THE
RESTLESS
VISIONARY

THE
RESTLESS
VISIONARY

HOW ONE MAN FOUND
HIMSELF, AND SPARKED
A WELLNESS REVOLUTION

Mel Zuckerman
FOUNDER, CANYON RANCH
And Louisa Kasdon

CANYON RANCH PRESS

Published by the Canyon Ranch Press
8600 East Rockcliff Road, Tucson, Arizona 85750 USA

Printed in the United States of America

Canyon Ranch is a registered trademark of
ZC Investments, LLC

www.canyonranch.com

Design by Canyon Ranch Inc.
Teri Bingham and Christopher Sahlin

Library of Congress Control Number: 2010942348

THE RESTLESS VISIONARY
How one man found himself, and sparked a wellness revolution

Zuckerman, Mel and Kasdon, Louisa

ISBN 978-0-9831844-0-9

To Enid

Dedicated to my loving wife, Enid.
Her vision permeated my soul.
Her support and trust defined my destiny.
Her unselfish and abundant generosity has given
more to me, to our family and to the world
than she can ever know.

CONTENTS

FOREWORD
By Dr. Andrew Weil

———————◆•◆•◆———————

Mel Zuckerman's vision for Canyon Ranch and the wellness revolution it inspired was sparked by the sudden insight that he could take control of his health and life and teach others to do the same. In this candid autobiography he relates how he came to that realization, how he acted on it to create a world-famous health resort, and how he has navigated the ups and downs of running a wellness empire for more than three decades. Now in his 80s, Mel is an inspiring example of healthy aging. Together with his wife, Enid, he continues to oversee the activities of Canyon Ranch and direct his energies and philanthropy toward improving public health, medicine and individual well-being.

I first met Mel a few years after the original Canyon Ranch opened in Tucson, my hometown. I worked with him to design a Natural Healing Department at the Ranch, which gave me a chance to develop the style of practice that I came to call Integrative Medicine and later began to teach at the University of Arizona College of Medicine.

Integrative Medicine focuses on the body's innate powers of self-healing and emphasizes prevention through attention to lifestyle. It is my passion and the focus of my professional life. I believe that it also represents the future of medicine and is a large part of the solution to the health care crisis that threatens our whole economy. Integrative Medicine can lower health care costs in two ways. First, by addressing the influences of lifestyle choices on health and disease risks, it can shift "health care" of today away from disease management toward real prevention and health promotion. Second, it can bring into the mainstream less expensive, low-tech treatments that can preserve or enhance health outcomes.

Mel Zuckerman was an early supporter of the Program in Integrative Medicine, now the Arizona Center for Integrative Medicine, a center of excellence at our university. Physician graduates of the center's fellowship training direct medical services at Canyon Ranch facilities. Early on, Mel and I saw that we were working for the same ends, and as we go forward I expect that we will continue to do so. One of my present academic titles—and one I am very proud to hold—is professor of public health at the Mel and Enid Zuckerman College of Public Health.

You will get to know Mel very well in these pages. I am sure that, like me, you will find the story of his life a compelling example of personal transformation and remarkable achievement and success—success based on inspiration, dedication, perseverance and hard work. Mel Zuckerman is indeed a visionary, and given his restless nature, I am sure he has not yet finished turning his vision into reality.

Tucson, Arizona
April, 2010

THE
RESTLESS
VISIONARY

The goal of life is to die young ... as late as possible
– Ashely Montagu, quoting ancient Greek philosophy

INTRODUCTION

On a sunny spring morning in 1978, my wife, Enid, and I first set foot on the land that is now Canyon Ranch. The place was a dilapidated dude ranch then, and the dusty road in was lined with tall eucalyptus trees, a rare stretch of shade that took us past a corral and some broken-down stables. The road ended at a small cluster of buildings, dry grass and cactus. Standing in front of the main ranch house, you could see the edges of the property, a tree-lined creek on one side and a couple of scrub and saguaro-covered hills, with the rough silhouette of the Santa Catalina Mountains in the distance. The ambience was part Old West, part sunbaked cheap motel, most everything falling down or gone to ruin.

But as we walked down a flagstone path near the sagging ranch house, both of us knew there was something there that was easy to miss if you focused just on the tumbleweeds and musty Jacuzzi. The eucalyptus trees along the creek were shining green, and the crags of Mount Lemmon stood out against a deep blue sky.

"Do you feel the magic?" That's what we said to each other.

Nothing about that place had said "magic" to anyone for a long, long time. But I could somehow feel the soul of the land, and sense what was possible there. An image flashed into my mind's eye that day—a vision of an oasis with the sound of water bubbling through, a place where people would come to change their lives. And as I look around now, 32 years later, that's what I see: a healing complex set in an oasis of a resort that spreads over a site four times larger than the original ranch. Fifteen thousand people find their way here every year to transform their bodies, minds and souls in ways that are often profound.

They may not arrive with the word transformation in mind. It could be that they're struggling with weight problems or an addiction or a grave health diagnosis and think we can help. They may just want to decompress and have fun on bike rides and hikes through the stark, magnificent landscape of the Sonoran Desert. Or sharpen up their golf game. But by the time they leave, they'll have been exposed to classes and lectures on fitness, health, metaphysics, art, sports and beauty. Perhaps they'll have encountered the innovative medical professionals in our Health & Healing Center, or found the tools for making lasting lifestyle changes at our

Life Enhancement Center. They may even have experienced therapies such as healing touch and Watsu from our nurses and body workers, or entered the world of shamanic journeying.

None of this would exist if someone hadn't looked at an unhappy and dangerously unhealthy guy, seen the resilient spirit buried in him and introduced him to a force he'd never before encountered: the power of possibility. I was that stressed-out, struggling guy. And I'm still amazed that the experience that transformed me—a visit to a "fat farm" in the late 1970s—inadvertently helped launch a wellness revolution.

When I read articles that describe me as a visionary, I have to laugh. I'm anything but. Deciding to build Canyon Ranch, I had no strategic plan, no grand aspirations and no sweeping idea for anything. I just knew one thing: I'd spent a month at a fat farm. And after a lifetime of believing that I'd never be truly well or comfortable in my body, I came away knowing that I had the power to make a lasting change in my health. "I want to feel this way forever," I told Enid.

When I saw that it could happen for me, I knew it could happen for others as well. I had found my mission: helping people with unhealthy lifestyles and restless souls make the transition to a healthier life.

The story that follows is the chaotic and crazy tale of how one imperfect, overweight, overstressed, often impulsive and irrational man woke up at 50, took a dramatic turn to wellness and never once looked back. I unearthed surprising possibilities in myself, and found a way to build a place—and then spark a movement—in which other people could do it too.

When I look back over the earliest letters I received from our guests at Canyon Ranch, I keep circling the words "magic," "miracle" and "nirvana." These are words that rarely pop up in the day-to-day conversations of the serious, worldly population we serve. Still, they are the words our guests, both first-timers and long-timers, continue to use. I flip through the new letters on my desk and they sound almost the same as those in my early files. "Miracle." "Nirvana." "Magic."

I believe it's there in the land in Tucson. But I've come to see that if you search for it out there somewhere—in the mesquite or among the mourning doves, quail and javelina that give so much character to the property—you'll miss it entirely. More than anything, I think that whatever magic people feel is actually the glimmer of possibility they discover inside themselves when they come to Tucson, or any of the Canyon Ranch properties. It's the amazing, resilient spirit they find in themselves. This book, and the years I have put into building Canyon Ranch, are dedicated to that spirit.

CHAPTER 1

Defining Moments

———◆•◆•◆———

For the first 50 years of my life, my body was my enemy, and I'm not sure I ever fully enjoyed a single day. I was just 8 years old when I got the strong message that if I weren't careful, my lungs would betray me. I'd been wheezing all night with an asthma attack, and my mother was in a panic. She had tried all the medicine in the house to help me breathe, and nothing worked. So in the early morning, she phoned our doctor. He met us in the emergency room at Hackensack Hospital in New Jersey just after dawn. Even though I was exhausted and struggling to take in air, the doctor made me giggle. He was about 5'2" tall and about 5'3" wide. He must have weighed 400 pounds, and he waddled when he walked. He had a little fringe around his bald head, horn-rimmed glasses perched on his nose and a stethoscope that he turned this way and that, listening as he tapped on my chest and back. After a few minutes, he went to his black bag, took out a syringe and filled it with adrenalin. He stood in front of me, poised to give me the shot. A cigarette dangled from his mouth, with just enough ash to fascinate me. Would it fall? Wouldn't it? As he plunged the needle into my left arm, he turned to my mother, took a puff, blew the smoke in my face, and said, "Mrs. Zuckerman, don't ever let Melvin exercise, because if he exercises, he'll get sick."

For an 8-year-old, that was a death sentence. Exercise was another word for everything kids called play. But it was 1936, a time when the doctor was God—even one who was a walking advertisement for a heart attack. And our doctor was actually right in step with the prevailing thinking in the 1930s that exercise induced asthma. My mother, always anxious and overprotective of her only child, clung to those words and watched me like a hawk to enforce them. There would be no gym classes, no running with the other kids on the block after school. When all the rest of the guys were outside on bikes, or playing stickball on the street, I'd be home alone, reading.

The truth was, any time I tried to exercise, I did get sick, wheezing and pale. My parents were petrified, and so was I. I became miserable, lonely and introverted. I lived with an endless list of things I couldn't do. There was no schoolyard baseball, or football, or basketball for little Melvin. I was the anxious kid who had to stand by and watch while the other guys ran around and played. I got used to living with lots of don'ts: Don't do this; don't do that, or you'll get sick. Slowly but surely, I became a boy who was afraid that almost everything I attempted would hurt me. On the rare occasions that I was allowed out to the park to play baseball, or when I snuck out through a window, I was afraid that if I hit more than a single I'd be wheezing so hard by the time I got on base I'd have to race home to inhale my medicine from a large glass atomizer. I didn't learn to ride a bike until I was almost 11. And for decades, I felt sidelined by my body.

When I discovered almost 50 years later that I could play sports, even run a marathon, and have fun doing all sorts of physical things, my whole world opened up. But in those early years I was always protecting myself, shrinking back. It would be revolutionary to discover in the middle of my life that exercise was my road to wellness, health and vitality.

Anxious, but dreaming

There's not much I like to remember about my childhood. Illness and restriction had defined my life even before I got the "no exercise" sentence. I feared everything new. When I started kindergarten, I threw up every single day. Nervous, insecure and uncomfortable in my own skin, I worried about everything. But in that, I was my parents' child. My father, Norman Zuckerman, struggled to support us during the Depression. He owned a paint and wallpaper store in Hackensack but he didn't have the patience to deal with the women who'd come in, deliberating over which color blue would look best in their kitchens and whether they wanted flowers or geometrics. He depended on my mother to go in and handle the fussy customers, but even then the business wasn't a huge success—and it was only the latest in a long line of dismal attempts to make a go of things.

My father had gone in and out of business five times by the time we moved to Hackensack, and each business failure had meant another move, a deeper hole. There were days when he would lift me up to the cash register in the paint store and show me the lines of zeroes. My parents were consumed by money worries, arguing loudly and constantly. My mother, Shirley Zuckerman, was unsatisfied. She wanted to do things, or to buy things, or go places, as any other woman might. But there was no money for indulging her wishes. My father would listen as long as he could, and then he'd put an end to the conversation by losing his temper, pounding on the table and telling her to just "Shut up!" Affection and peace were scarce commodities at home.

My mother coped by staying tethered to her friends, with whom she pored over every detail of our life and theirs. When she came home from the store, she'd pop her head into my bedroom to check on me, and then go downstairs to prepare dinner. The sound that rose from the kitchen, louder than the chopping and sizzling, was a steady stream of conversation. She'd call her best friend, Hattie, then move on to her next best friends, Nettie and Sophie. And if she had time, she'd call Esther. Dinner was served when the last friend hung up.

Mom was also the family perfectionist—that is, she wanted me to be perfect. Although she had an upbeat, positive outlook on most things, she was tough on me, much tougher than my dad. If I brought home a report card that had four "E's" for excellent and one "G" for good, all we ever talked about was the lone "G" and why it wasn't an "E." But I have to admit that she motivated me to succeed, to work harder, to be—and seek—the best.

My dad was mostly concerned with putting one foot in front of the other and trying to keep going. The glass was always three-quarters empty for him. Even as a boy, I suspected that there was something wrong with him. Today, I'd say that he was chronically depressed, but I didn't know those kinds of words then. What I did know was that when your father leaves the store every afternoon because he has to take a nap, something is very wrong. No one else's dad did that. Yet he was a sweet, caring man—and a fabulous whistler. His favorite tunes were Christmas carols, and for the whole month of December he'd whistle them, especially "Silent Night," a funny choice for a thoroughly Jewish man. No matter what the money situation, he took me to the movies every Saturday morning. Once or twice a year, he would take my friends and me to baseball games at Ebbets Field in Brooklyn or the Polo Grounds in Manhattan. When we got older, there were excursions to the circus and movies in New York City. I think it was his escape from business pressures and my mother, as well as his best shot at being a loving dad.

I carried legacies from both my parents—my father's caring, humility and depression, my mother's drive and perfectionism—when I stepped out of their world into my own life. I'd also found something all my own: daydreaming. With my parents preoccupied with business and survival, and the outside world of street games and fun off-limits to me, I actually enjoyed going to bed early because I could escape into my own little fantasy world. I'd imagine myself as Dick Tracy, the detective from the funny pages, catching the bad guys with my little stub revolver. Radio serials like "The Adventures of Jack Armstrong, the All-American Boy" and "Captain Midnight" became favorites of mine too.

Following the local sports teams, especially the Brooklyn Dodgers, was my other outlet. I'd sit in the living room in front of the big old Philco radio, listening to Red Barber announcing the Dodgers' games from Ebbets Field. He was broadcasting right from the field, and you could hear all the fans, with the catcalls and the hoots, along with the sounds of the players on the field. The Dodgers were known as "dem bums." Just like that: d – e – m bums, because they'd never won anything since 1918. But we loved them, with their colorful players, nicknamed things like Mickey, Dixie, Cookie and Ducky. But, boy! I remember such teen anguish when they lost that I kicked in the screen door. Even as a child I had an impressive temper.

Mostly, though, I remember looking out of the windows a lot and daydreaming. Occasionally I wonder if all that time spent rooting for underdogs, listening to adventures where risks always paid off and the good guys always won—prepared me well for a life where I was willing to risk everything, time and time again.

The lessons of a brand-new bike

Like all kids, I wanted a bike. All the other boys in the neighborhood already had them, and they would ride to school in the mornings, then circle the block in a two-wheeler gang after school, while I was left sitting cross-legged on my stoop. By age 10 I was bugging and bugging and bugging my mother, "Why can't I have a bike?" But she wasn't listening. Finally, my friends took up my cause. A group of guys from the block literally got on their knees in front of my mom and pleaded with her. Until then, my father hadn't paid any attention to the discussion, but after that visit, it was, "OK, let's go look for one." So, on a Saturday morning, he and I went over to Pep Boys. In the window was a beautiful 26-inch bike. Red and white, brand-new and shiny. My tongue was hanging out. It was everything a 10-year-old boy could ever want in a bike. The price tag in the window read "$19.95." My father said, "We'll think about it." And we walked out of the store in total silence.

For the next two or three days, like a typical kid, I pestered him for his decision. Finally, he turned to me and said very quietly, "Mel, I just can't afford it." I could see how hard it was for him to spit it out. OK. I got it. No shiny red and white bike. I also understood that my father was ashamed in front of me.

I wasn't ready to give up on the idea of getting a bike, though. Without telling anyone, I took a walk to a shop that sold used bikes. It had this old yellow one. It wasn't shiny, but it was a bike and the price tag read $7.

A day or so later, I said to my father, "Let's go look at this other bike store."

"Mel, they're even more expensive than Pep Boys," he said.

"I saw a bicycle in the window that I think is OK."

My dad, with sad, sad eyes, said, "OK, we'll go have a look."

We went to the store and I pointed out the bike. It was old, and someone had repainted it. More or less. Gamely, I took it out to the sidewalk and rode it a little bit, and then I wheeled it back and said, "Dad, I love it!"

"Wait a minute," my father said. He got down on his hands and knees and started inspecting it closely, running his finger over the fenders. He found a little dent that had been painted over with yellow paint. With a hint of tears that were unmistakable even to a child, he said, "You know, the price is good. But I just don't want to buy you a damaged bike."

I said, "No, Dad. It's really perfect."

"No, it isn't," he said.

I did my best not to show how dejected I was. The next day after school he said to me, "Let's go over to Pep Boys." He signed a note to pay $2 a month for three years. That was $72 total—for a $20 bike. It was as clear a proof of his love for me as there could ever be. And it established the sense in me that a man needs to feel the pride of providing material things for his family—even if the cost, from the outside, seems extravagantly high.

The world gets a little bigger

I started working fairly young. Like everyone else I knew, if I wanted money for a milkshake or a movie, I had to earn it myself. As a 14-year-old, I started delivering telegrams for Western Union. It was 1942, during World War II, and I found myself carrying "star" telegrams from the Army to the homes of families whose sons and husbands were dead or missing in action. Even before I got to the door the recipients were already hysterical. I couldn't take it. And believe me, you don't get a 10-cent tip from a mother who has just learned that her son is missing in action. I quit after four months. Next I worked as a stock clerk, in the basement of a wholesale drug store, opening boxes and putting things on the shelves. Hard, menial labor. In college, I clerked at a men's clothing store. Working—and the bike—made me feel self-sufficient. But that didn't add up to happiness. I was self-conscious about my appearance, uncomfortable in my skinny body and ill at ease being a Jewish kid in a very non-Jewish neighborhood during World War II. I was haunted by the feeling that I was somehow "less than" the other boys.

But I could transport myself into imagined places and see possibilities that were invisible to most people. And eventually—though it took half a lifetime—I could even see them in myself.

CHAPTER 2

Goodbye to the Shy Boy

———◆◆◆◆———

When I was 14, we moved to our first house. In many ways it was a step up: a home of our own instead of a rental. But things were cramped. A one-bathroom, two-story, it had three bedrooms on the second floor. One was mine, one was my parents', and the third one was occupied by my two grandmothers. From the old country, neither grandmother spoke English, and one was ill most of the time and never left her room. I suppose that it was their coming to live with us that motivated my parents to buy a house. A tiny fourth room was rented out to a boarder. It was a financial stretch even then to buy an old house for $4,000.

By that time, much of my life was school, my after-school jobs and my friends. "Girls" were still just an idea. For all my shyness, I had the best friends, not a lot of them—three or four. We've remained close for our entire lives, maybe because all of us were from the wrong side of the tracks. Literally. We all lived within two or three blocks of one another, just a couple of blocks from the railroad tracks. We loved to play ball, and sometimes I would let myself out of my bedroom window with a sheet tied to the bedpost and meet them at the park. I was slight but tough. When we played football at the park, I was the fullback because nobody could ever drag me down. Always very competitive, I would have liked to go out for a sport in high school, but I settled for being the best ping-pong player at Hackensack High. Ping-pong didn't have the hoopla of high school football or baseball, but it didn't aggravate my asthma. Unfortunately, though, being a table tennis champ (instead of a "real" tennis champ) didn't do much to give me a sense of confidence in my body.

A lot of the male ego is wrapped up in physicality, and physical prowess affects a man's perception of his worth and sexuality. It seems that no amount of career success can entirely balance the scale when a guy feels like a physical zero. I understand that because I lived it as a teenager and young man. I was a better than decent student, mostly because I was one of those kids who was always nervous that he'd fail the test. My memory was good—I could practically visualize the page in the textbook—and I could usually depend on it to get me through the exam. I wasn't brilliant, but I worked hard and performed well enough that my teachers always encouraged me to think about college.

Even so, I was an insecure wreck, and I was sure that no matter how bright I was, I wasn't attractive to women. As much as I wanted to be one of the guys shooting hoops or banging home runs, I also wanted to score with the girls. But I was so afraid to put my arm around a girl, so afraid that the girl would reject me, that I would never make a move. It's funny. When I look back at photos of myself as a teenager and young man, I wasn't bad looking at all. I'd developed a big, deep chest and a good physique—both with no effort— but I carried around that image of Mel as a skinny, runty kid as if it were my permanent ID card.

I was madly in love with a 14-year-old girl when I was 16. The first time we went to a movie together, she reached over to take my hand and placed it on her shoulder. Like a dummy, I sat frozen—I couldn't imagine what I was supposed to do next. But she was persistent, and placed my hand lightly on her breast. Here was a younger girl trying to lead me, the "older" man, through a process of what to do when you are sitting next to a girl at a movie on a "date." And I was clueless. My fingers didn't massage or caress or casually edge—they just sat there. Later, I learned that she had confided in my next-door neighbor, "You know, I like him a lot, but I can't get anywhere with Mel." I can honestly admit that this was the only time in my life when I didn't take advantage of a good opportunity.

For all my friends and my good work at school, teen

angst hit me hard. I was nervous about going to college, even though I'd just be commuting across the river to NYU and living at home. The idea of having to start again and make new friends, now that I was separated from my little clique from junior high school and high school, scared me. Doors were opening wide and I was afraid to walk through. But I was more afraid not to.

A conversation with myself

In the first few days of college, I knew I had to come out of my shell. Waiting for the subway one evening, I had a talk with myself. "Do you want college to be four more miserable years? Or do you want to try to do something different?" I asked the withdrawn Mel I'd been. "Is this what you want your life and future to be? Or do you want to try to manifest a different personality?" And I remember thinking, "This new personality may not be you, but it might get you more of what you want from life." I was determined to be more outgoing, take more risks and be a little flirtatious and forward with women, even though it was a struggle for me.

I remember challenging myself, talking to myself as if I were my own best friend. "So, Mel, you've completed your first week of college, and what did you do? You hid. It doesn't have to be this way. You do have time to be social, to meet people, to be more outgoing. You've got time in between class; you can get there early or stay late and figure out how to become part of the college community." The next day, I forced myself to go into the main student lounge and decided to learn to play chess. I sat and sat, watching the other guys play. After a few weeks, I joined them, and I was pretty good. I started to make friends. It was a deliberate, conscious decision to reinvent myself and leave behind the miserable, limited world I'd felt stuck in since childhood.

I worked on my personality as if it were a school project. I became more gregarious, sometimes to the point of being assertive. During those four years, from 18 to 22, I was diligent in developing my social skills. I learned to fake it, to act more confident, to be more outspoken. To be the guy with the fastest quips. In photos of myself from those years, I can see that I was projecting that confidence too. I'm not saying it was all for the better, because as I look back, I realize that I pushed away my sensitive, quiet side. But the outgoing persona had begun to work. I was finally getting happy. Being more confident, I decided, was a lot better than being shy.

But I wasn't outspoken enough at that point to challenge my parents, who had decreed that I would enter the job market as an accountant since I excelled in math. From the first, I knew I was going to hate it, and I did, but they insisted. They pointed out that I had two cousins who were accountants and they were "doing well." Besides, how many choices did a kid from a poor family have in those days? As much as I wanted to go away to school, to someplace exotic, the reality was that, at least for a while, I needed to live at home, commute to New York and learn my way around a balance sheet. The bizarre thing is, I was good at it. And I couldn't imagine where I'd get the money to do something else.

Meeting Enid

After graduating, I was restless. I took a job at the accounting office where I had worked part time in college, but I knew it wasn't for me and I quit in a few months. Then I tried a few months of working in the paint and wallpaper store with my father. The good news was that I realized there was something I hated more than accounting! I tried my luck reinventing myself in Florida, but that didn't last either, and I found myself back in New Jersey, back in accounting. I knew I was lucky to have a job and a steady paycheck.

With a little money in my pocket, I began to date. When I was introduced to Enid Slotkin on a blind date in November '52, it just worked. She was a cute, redheaded dental hygienist, and we laughed at the same jokes. From the first night we felt comfortable and had fun with each other, and we quickly slipped into the sense that our futures would be entwined. Her parents liked me. My parents adored her. She was a bit younger, but I was hardly more mature.

Seven months later, we were married and living in a $72-a-month apartment, with friends and family around.

I yearned for a different career, but I was happy with my life and my wife. There was just one small red flag beginning to wave. Early in our marriage, when Enid and I would argue (what couple doesn't?), that temper I'd had as a kid would rear up. She'd get fearful and I'd apologize, a difficult dance we'd do again and again through our marriage. The sensitive kid I'd tried to get rid of was gone, all right, and we were seeing the first signs he'd left a tougher, angrier man behind.

CHAPTER 3

The Adventure Begins

———◆•◆•◆———

I've always been a restless soul—maybe all unhappy people are. It's been part of my drive for perfection and growth—that feeling of never being satisfied wherever I am, the appetite for more. I'd always had this idea that my future wasn't in New Jersey but somewhere in the West. When one of my friends from the old neighborhood moved to the Bay Area after college, I went out to visit. I was 21. What struck me were the people. Calm, kind, polite, friendly—they were the opposite of the pushy Easterners I'd grown up with. Maybe it was just me, but in the Bay Area, the taxicabs didn't try to run you down when you crossed the street. People actually slowed down to let you cross. I wanted to move there as soon as I could. But we stayed put in Hackensack and Enid got pregnant with our son Jay. We settled into our life as a young family.

For a lot of people, that would've been enough. I had a beautiful wife, and my first child was a boy, which should've been enough for any Jewish father. There were even rumors about making me a partner at the CPA firm. That was all the more remarkable because there had been a glut of accountants after World War II. The GI Bill made it possible for all the returning soldiers to go to college, and the shortest route to a secure profession for a veteran was to go to business school and become an accountant. As a non-veteran who'd gotten out of college just eight years earlier, I knew in 1950 I had been lucky to get a job making $20 a week as a junior accountant. That was 50 cents an hour for a 40-hour week. Now eight years later I was secure, and rising fast.

But I hated what I was doing. I spent my days with numbers and corporate tax returns instead of people. I accepted that it was my responsibility to put bread on the table for my family, especially now that I had a son, but I was never going to find happiness as a CPA in Hackensack. I had a serious case of get-me-out-of-New Jersey.

I'd been trying to get Enid to go west ever since our honeymoon in '53. When I suggested California, she said, "What for? Why would we want to go all the way across the country when there are so many beautiful places so much closer? And money is so tight."

So we took a car trip to Niagara Falls and to Canada, like everyone else we knew. I mentioned my fantasy of living out West someday, but that didn't fly either. Enid made it immediately clear she wasn't moving away from her family. Period.

I didn't give up, though. I'd mention the idea periodically, and brace myself for the answer: "It ain't gonna happen. Out of the question." But it's funny how things can change. In January 1958, Enid decided to go with her parents on their yearly visit to see her sister, Bernice, who now lived in Yuma, Arizona. Jay was 3, and he seemed to catch every ear, nose and throat bug as soon as the weather changed, so Enid was taking him with her, hoping that a winter in the desert would build him up enough that he could get his tonsils out. Jay flourished in the warm weather—and Enid had a change of heart.

In January, Yuma is beautiful. Hot and dry, it's everything that winter isn't in New Jersey. Enid loved it. She called me from her sister's. "You know that idea about moving West? I think I'm ready." I was thrilled. We made the decision right away. "That's how we did things in those days," Enid likes to tease me. "We were never planners." How right she is. We've always moved on our instincts. For better or worse.

Enid came home in March and we started planning for the move. It somehow didn't matter to us that she was pregnant again, or that our life savings was just $1,800. We'd point ourselves toward the Pacific and see what happened. California seemed like our best bet. I'd seen a want ad in the Journal of Accountancy from a CPA who wanted to find a younger partner to take over his practice in Santa Monica. And the friend who had lured me West in the first place was now a CPA in San Francisco. He was begging me to join him so we could start our own accounting firm. That was my ace in the hole. I'd see what other options turned up, but at least I had one solid opportunity. If being a CPA in Jersey was hell, maybe being a CPA in California would just be purgatory— or better. Who knew? Well anyway, we were headstrong and probably irrational. It was time for an adventure.

I gave my notice, we gave up our apartment, and we sold everything that wouldn't fit in our car. As Enid remembers, there wasn't much to dispose of. We were young, and hadn't the means or the time to acquire a lot of "stuff." So we set off in the summer, with Enid and Jay in the front seat and our suitcases and boxes in the back. We planned to drive all over the West and the Southwest, and up and down the coast of California. We'd take our time, and it would be a vacation, except that we weren't going home. The bets all over New Jersey were that I'd be back within six months. "You'll never be able to stay away." "You'll be back, you'll be back, you'll be back." But as far as I was concerned, we were through with the East. This move was forever.

I planned the route carefully and made reservations for every night based on the distance I thought we'd travel that day in our brand-new 1958 Nash Rambler. The days were long. We got lost in Nebraska, and poor Enid got carsick as we crossed the Rockies, a stomach-turning blur of switchbacks that didn't sit well in early pregnancy. One day, after we'd been in the car for 13 hours, she slept in the bathtub to be next to the toilet.

This was before freeways and parkways, and certainly before GPS's. I got on the wrong road and Enid said, "Just stop over there and ask directions." But I was too stubborn. It's one of my weaknesses. But then again, if I didn't have a stubborn determination, Canyon Ranch would never have been born—or survived.

We loved California. Loved each place we visited more than the last. And in each place we stopped—the Bay Area, Santa Monica, San Diego—I had a job offer. But before we could decide where to settle, we wanted to visit Enid's sister and her family in Yuma.

Arizona might be lovely in January, but this was August, and the closer we got, the more extreme the conditions. When we stopped to get something to eat in El Centro, California, not far from the Arizona border, the crickets were so thick on the restaurant's floor they crunched underfoot when you walked. It was so hot that you'd singe your hand when you touched the windshield, and you didn't dare touch the handle on the outside of the car door with a bare hand. When we finally arrived in Yuma an hour and a half later, it was 117 degrees. At 9:30 p.m.

Enid was so exhausted she wanted to turn around and go back to California. But I told her that as soon as we got to her sister's house, the air conditioning and the rest would revive her and Jay. We'd been on the road for six weeks, and now she was almost five months pregnant. I settled the two of them in and went to scout out the territory like a cowboy out of an old Western. I headed for Phoenix, where once again I was offered a job, and then went on to Tucson.

In those days, Tucson was like a little Old West town, with maybe 100,000 people living in an enormous valley surrounded by mountains. When I first drove in, I thought, "Whoa! Do they still tie the horses in front of the stores?" But it was love at first sight. I loved the weather (supposedly good for people with asthma), the mountains and the canyons, and the fact that it was a university town likely to draw an interesting community as it grew. I said to myself, "This is where I was meant to be." I felt a spiritual pull to the place, although spiritual isn't a word I would have used then. Tucson sang to me.

After a few days of looking around town, I hadn't found a job. But for some reason, that didn't bother me. I called Enid, who told me she was ready to "head right back to California." It hardly registered. "I'm coming to get you and bringing you to Tucson," I said.

"What for?" she said, distraught. "Tucson is a desert! I'm a city girl! I can't live in a cow town!"

It was probably an irrational decision, but I was determined to plant my family next to the Santa Catalina Mountains.

Phoenix would've suited Enid better. It had tall buildings and enough amenities to satisfy a girl who was used to getting to Times Square in 20 minutes on the train. But I was resolute—maybe even a little mean—and Enid gave in. It was the '50s, and she knew that I'd have to be the one to earn a living, so the choice of where to do it was mine. She'd raise the kids, and she knew she'd find friends among the other young families. But Tucson was never where she wanted to be.

We moved into a motel and I scoured the town for jobs. But three weeks later, I was still empty-handed. Much to Enid's delight, we got back in the car and started back for the West Coast. But since we needed to go north before cutting over to the California border, I suggested we drive through Phoenix so she could take a look. The bigger city appealed to her enough that she said she was willing to try living there— it was no Manhattan, but it was better than Tucson!

I thought it might work. California seemed too life-in-the-fast-lane to me and I wasn't a fast-lane type of guy in 1958 (I'm still not). So we decided to give Phoenix a few days and called our Tucson motel to give them our forwarding address. A phone message was waiting: An accountant in Tucson had been trying to reach me. His partner had decided to go off on his own, and the office urgently needed a senior CPA. I turned the car right around.

The truth is that Enid cried for 20 years. But for me, from the moment I drove in off Miracle Mile, Tucson was my home. And eventually it became the place where our great adventure—Canyon Ranch—began.

CHAPTER 4

Riding the Real Estate
Roller Coaster

———◆•◆•◆———

I n retrospect, I think of the 1960s and my own 30s and
40s as "my anxious years." Within months of our move
to Tucson, I had abandoned my safe, dependable career
as a CPA and launched myself as a home builder. Those
were the years I learned about risk.

With a loan from our parents, Enid and I bought our first
house two weeks after we arrived. Our daughter, Amy, was
due in just a few months. I dutifully went to my new job in
the accounting office, but I told my new boss on the day he
hired me that he shouldn't plan on my staying with him for
the long run.

Having made one big break with my past, I was on the
hunt for the next. One of our clients at the accounting firm had
a small real estate and insurance brokerage business, and over
lunch one day I asked him, "If you were a young guy starting

out in Tucson, where would you see the best opportunity?" He chewed for a minute and replied, "The way Tucson is growing ... I think the brightest future is in real estate."

Not long after, Enid and I went to a community gathering for new families, and I met a guy named Jack Young, who had been a real estate developer and home builder in Detroit. When I told him I was a CPA, he said, "Hmm, I've always had a CPA working for me." He offered me a job, and I figured it would be a good place to learn the real estate business close up.

I liked Jack, and I liked the work. I thought of it as sort of an internship. From the day I started, I was intent on learning the business. I took initiative and came in at night to work as he and his architects went over designs for new houses. They let me sit in on meetings, and every day I learned something new. I soaked up the details as he put his development together from the ground up. Jack liked me, and soon I was his right-hand man. Quickly, perhaps too quickly, I felt ready to try my hand at a real estate development of my own.

I was 31, energized and ambitious. One day I walked into Jack's office and said, "Jack, what's my future here?" I'd been working for him for only 18 months.

He said, "You know, I like you, and I think you've got a lot of ability but I haven't even thought about your future yet."

Overly cocky, I said, "Well, I need to think about it."

Jack was taken aback. "What do you need to think about?"

"Candidly," I said, "I have an offer to go in with somebody

else and start a building business." It was true. Someone was always talking about teaming up and going out on our own.

Jack got irritated and lit up a cigarette. "You'd be making a mistake," he said.

"Why?"

"Because you're not ready," he said, turning away and ending the conversation. That was like waving a red flag in front of me. I'd show him who was ready.

Leap and learn

It was 1960, and Tucson was growing rapidly, with big employers like Hughes Aircraft and Martin Marietta hiring heavily and attracting young families to the area. How could I miss? Real estate development worked for me. I got the hang of it quickly, and I put my 18 months of on-the-job training with Jack to good use. This new vocation called on all sorts of natural talents that I didn't suspect I had. I liked the action and rhythm: lots of meetings, driving around to sites, working with contractors, bankers, architects and public officials. Much higher energy than sitting in an office as an accountant, making columns of numbers talk back to me.

I was a new man, and I needed a new personality— something a little tougher and more suitable for the construction world. I was straightforward and fair in my dealings, but I used that temper of mine to get the contractors to meet my standards of quality and perfection. From my father I had learned that if you pounded your hand hard enough on the table and bellowed loud enough, it usually stopped the conversation. Some contractors would try to take advantage of the numbers guys who spent time working in their offices, assuming they knew little about construction. But they soon knew better than to try that with me. More than once, I pushed out my chest into a guy's chest, stuck out my finger and said, "You'll do it my way." I backed down more contractors than I can count. Partly they retreated because I scared them and partly because as the builder, I controlled their living. Most important: I paid on time and would advance them cash when they needed it. I liked my power, but I always played fair.

I found that I delighted in crafting all the elements of a successful real estate project, and I could see that my accounting background gave me a tremendous advantage over other small builders. In addition to easily mastering the numbers, I learned that I thoroughly enjoyed managing all aspects of the home-building business—thinking about everything from permits to water resources to design, finance and marketing issues. It turned out that I even liked selling, because I loved dealing with my customers. When families told me that moving into a home I'd built had transformed their lives, I was thrilled. It was as if I'd been doing it for years. Even though the stress was high—it's quite a leap from CPA to real estate developer—for the first time in my life, I loved what I was doing for a living.

Innovation at work, crisis
(then healing) at home

In 1960, I bought my first little parcel of land. Ten acres with an option to buy 10 more the following year, and 15 more later on. Tucson was still a hick town, but even so, there was a lot of competition among builders offering small 1,000- to 1,200-square-foot homes that could sell in the $9,000 to $12,000 range. My idea was to do something different, to make a home built by Mel Zuckerman a cut above the rest. I decided to take a chance, and I bought land to build on that was on the wrong side of town, but within the best school district in Tucson. My gamble paid off. The houses at Harmony Homes sold quickly, and my first project was a success. I was beginning to garner respect as a builder and businessman, and I fantasized about having enough money in the bank to retire at 40; the way things were going, nothing seemed out of reach. I also liked being considered an innovator as a developer. I was the pioneer who built the first recreation center in a development at my price point, and the first one to offer high quality finishes in the most modest homes. I had always itched to be creative, ahead of the curve, and now I was leading the pack in both ingenuity and integrity.

In 1961, just as I was getting started with a new housing subdivision, Enid was diagnosed with a melanoma in her thigh. "She could die from this," the doctor said. "We're going to have to do surgery, and probably the best outcome is amputating her leg above the thigh." Enid was terrified and I was scared for all of us. Jay was 5 and Amy was only 2. The operation seemed to go on forever, and when the doctor finally came into the waiting room I fainted. But the news was good: They'd been able to remove the cancerous area and save her leg. Thank God! I was overcome with relief and full of love for my wife. But as soon as she was out of danger, I drove right back to work. Where else would I go?

Fears about Enid's health hovered for the next five years, and she responded by changing her life, reading health and nutrition books and paying attention to what she ate and how much exercise she got. She intuited that by keeping her body healthy, she could keep the cancer at bay. Me? I didn't intuit anything; I just stuffed my anxieties and plowed everything I had into my business.

I'd sold out my first two subdivisions as well as two apartment complexes that I built simultaneously, and by 1962 I was able to make the down payment of $200,000 and sign a note for $1 million to buy a big parcel of land that I decided to call Sabino Vista, in the northeast corner of the county. I'd come a long way from making $150 a week as an accountant, and I seemed to have a golden touch. Now I was thinking big. My mood was up, I was confident, and we had a lot of friends.

Now an experienced home builder, I built my family

a beautiful new house, double the size of our first home in Tucson. It was set on a four-acre lot with terrific mountain views of the Santa Catalinas. We had a beautiful big backyard with a swimming pool and a large fenced-in dog run. I remember looking at my new address, thinking, "What a great place to raise my family."

But fatherhood did not come easily to me. I wanted to be the model all-American dad but nothing in my upbringing had prepared me for the emotional challenges of parenting. Fortunately, Enid was a natural parent, a great mom and advocate for our two kids. When I look back at those years with my young family, I see so many lost opportunities. I wish as a father that I had been more present and less overwrought.

At the time, though, it all seemed magical to me. Such an improvement over my own childhood in New Jersey! We had bunnies on the porch and a cluster of dogs and puppies running around the yard. House, backyard, swimming pool, dogs, kids—that piece of my life seemed in order. We took occasional family vacations to the beach, and when we were home, we'd sit in the family room and watch "Star Trek" and other TV shows together. I thought we were the typical American family growing up in the '60s.

I taught both kids to swim in our backyard pool. I do have one regret: Whenever I'd race Jay in the pool, I'd touched the wall before he did. I should have let him win once in a while. I thought it would make him reach harder, swim faster, but in retrospect, it was a mistake for me to beat him time after time. Given what I'd learned from my mother, I thought parenting was all about getting your kids to reach for perfection. How many times over the years have I wished for a second chance at parenthood!

When I had time on the weekends, I'd go horseback riding with the kids. Amy became besotted with horses. At 6, she was brushing the horses in the stables at the Sabino Vista Recreation Center. I bought Jay a horse, and the two of us rode together in the parade for the Tucson Rodeo. Jay's horse reared up—Amy and Enid were watching from the sidelines—and everyone cheered as Jay managed to control the horse. I also loved being his Little League coach. Jay was one of the smaller kids on the team and I doubted he'd ever get a chance to play. But the kids surprised me. When I gave them the choice of making sure we won every game, or making sure everyone got to play, they chose "playing all" over "winning all." I was proud of my team, and I think I was a pretty good coach.

Family life was good when business was good. But the warm fuzzy turned abrasive when my business ran into difficulty. When things got rough at the office, the wear and tear was evident at home. No time, no patience, no emotional support. Those were the bad years, and even though we've all made peace with how our family was, the kids still bear the emotional scars of an angry father, terrified of becoming a failure.

Developing Sabino Vista

The plan was to build 60 to 100 homes a year on the 400 acres of Sabino Vista, a subdivision that would ultimately have 700 to 800 homes and would be served by a 25-acre recreation center with a pool, horse stabling and riding facilities, a clubhouse and tennis courts. This was a new market for Tucson—doctors, lawyers and other professionals—and it was a gamble. Our houses would sell for $20,000 to $30,000 in an area where the average mass-produced home went for $11,000 and everything over $15,000 was considered a "custom home."

Since I knew I couldn't compete directly with all the larger tract builders active in the Tucson market, I thought I'd have the best chance if I kept the focus on high-end quality. When people came into my homes, they would see the wow factor. Fancier kitchens and bathrooms. Nicer finishes. I leaned on Enid's taste to guide us—we were building for people like us, and our friends. "We shouldn't build anything that we wouldn't want to live in ourselves," she'd say as she selected the materials to put the finishing touches on our model homes. "No, this countertop is too cheap. These cabinets are too cheap. I'd never be satisfied with that in my own home." As a result, our houses "showed" nicer. Top quality, not minimalistic.

We built our houses better and priced them a little higher than the competition, quality over quantity. I never built more houses than I could visit every week during construction. Before I'd go to the office in the morning, I'd meet with the superintendent at each construction site. We really could never have more than 20 or 30 houses under construction at a time. I just didn't have enough hours in the day, or days in the week. Five or six was the most I could get through in the early morning. Though I started out with one partner and later added a second, from the first days of the business to the last, I was responsible for the day-to-day management of the company and the developments underway.

The perfectionism drilled into me by my mother was something I never learned to turn off. That meant a lot of angst for my contractors and suppliers.

In 1962, the state of Arizona required builders to extend a one-year warranty on a new home. I offered my buyers a five-year warranty. I wanted people to know that I'd stand behind the houses I'd built. I had a full-time construction, jack-of-all-trades handyman in a van circulating through my developments. His sole job was to go around and fix things. A door fell off its hinges, a window jammed or a leak developed in a plumbing line? No problem, the homeowner called the office and we took care of it—no matter how much time had elapsed, even if it wasn't strictly part of our warranty.

I enjoyed having direct contact with my customers. I'd sit with them as they picked out tile for the floors and the finishes for the cabinets. If they weren't totally happy with the styles or choices we had in our offices, we'd get in my car and go out to the distributor.

Bad news and more bad news

But quality and customer service alone couldn't insulate us from the ups and downs of the economy. We rode in on a boom, but in 1962, Martin Marietta laid off 1,500 employees. Then in late summer 1963, just as we put the first Sabino Vista homes on the market, Hughes Aircraft lost its government contract and cut 4,000 jobs. It was terrible news for a city our size, and doubly troubling for my business. When the company transferred its workers, it bought back their houses, flooding the market with homes for sale at prices I couldn't compete with. Worse, the layoffs decimated the ranks of the highly skilled professionals I'd hoped to lure at Sabino Vista.

The good news was that I wasn't stuck with a lot of unsold houses. On the other hand, I wasn't building enough new ones, and there was still a $1-million mortgage to pay on all those acres it now seemed foolish to develop. Just like my parents, I was consumed with financial worries and scrambling to stay afloat.

My personal life was unraveling. Being the engine behind Sabino Vista meant I was out of the house at first light, and rarely back before dark. It was hard to feel the closeness we'd had when Jay and Amy were small and I'd had time to enjoy our life together. And with the stresses building up, I was unleashing my temper as a matter of course on my job. I couldn't seem to rein it in at home either. Enid and I would go at each other regularly, and the kids had a ringside seat. They were scared of me.

Often after one of my outbursts, I'd be contrite and say to Enid, "That wasn't really me. I'm not my behavior. and I hope you know me well enough to know that." But she'd answer, "All I'm seeing is your behavior and not the sensitive, humble man you profess to be." She was right. Too often my behavior was intolerable, and it took me years to get the balance right.

My body was showing the strain. I was putting on weight and I had ulcers, high blood pressure and gastric issues. Although I'd first been diagnosed with high blood pressure as a teenager, by the time I was 40, my systolic blood pressure would rocket between 160 and 180, and my diastolic between 90 and 110. That's high. None of my conditions was a killer, but taken as a whole I was a pretty sick guy— a walking time bomb.

Stress relief for me involved food. I was working 10 to 12 hours a day, and I came home exhausted. After I ate dinner and kissed the kids goodnight, I'd read the paper for a while and put on the "boob tube." I was bored stiff, which was a problem. When you aren't particularly interested in the program on TV, and you have nothing to do with your hands, what do you do? You eat.

My drug of choice was Carnation Rocky Road ice cream, which I kept in a horizontal freezer. When we first moved to Tucson, we were tight on money, and there was an ad on TV for a food plan. Remember those? They gave you a month's supply of meat and threw in the freezer for free. But the meat on the plan was too fatty for Enid, and she put her foot down. "I don't care what it costs us," she said. "We're going back to our regular butcher." So we cancelled the plan, but bought the freezer. The only thing in it was my Rocky Road.

Every night, almost like clockwork, I'd turn on the TV, boredom would hit and I'd pull out a fresh half-gallon. Over time, I developed a system. At first it involved leaving the carton on the counter and letting it thaw. Later, in the '70s I'd put the carton in the microwave for 20 seconds and then I'd open the door, turn the carton halfway around and give it another 20 seconds. I'd take out a tablespoon and start scooping around the edges. Those were the best. They were already nice and soft. I'd work toward the center and all of a sudden, the TV program I was watching became interesting! Mouthful by mouthful, I pushed the day's troubles a little farther away. But I had some restraint. I didn't let myself finish the whole carton. I'd notice I was scraping the bottom and my inner voice would say: "Zuckerman, you're such a pig. You're not really going to eat that whole half-gallon." And boom! The top would go on and the carton would go back in the freezer, with two measly spoonfuls melting at the bottom. By my logic, that meant I didn't eat the whole thing.

I'd finish off the carton when I woke at 2 a.m., convinced that the only way to get back to sleep was to have a glass of milk with some cookies. Cookies without ice cream? What's that about? So I'd take out the half-gallon and down the last couple of scoops. I rationalized that it was OK because it was a different 24-hour period. Then the inner voice would start again. "What a pig! You actually finished it." It happened every single night.

At 5'9", I weighed 200 pounds. If I wasn't quite obese, I was dangerously overweight, especially given my health conditions.

The economic busts kept deepening, and by 1968, I was on the verge of declaring bankruptcy. At age 39, I was reading the classified ads looking for a job, wondering if Hughes Aircraft was hiring accountants. Neither my partner nor I had drawn a salary for more than two years. We were living off our savings, which were shrinking fast.

Betrayal

That year I weathered the worst dirty dealing and double-cross of my life. Back in 1962, my partner, Saul Tobin, and I had signed the million-dollar mortgage on the Sabino Vista land, agreeing to pay it off in 10 annual installments. As security, we had to put up not only the land, but also the water company we were setting up to serve the area. We had been able to squeeze out the first two mortgage payments in 1963 and 1964, but by 1965, with jobs dried up, the economy was in the tank and there were simply too few sales to cover our loan obligations. We were at our wits' end—money going out and too little coming in the front door. Saul and I both had young families to feed, and we knew we were out of gas, saddled with a huge debt. The only choice we could see was to give the land back to the lenders and get on with our lives.

So in January 1966, Saul and I flew to Detroit for a summit meeting with the original landowners. "This recession is really hurting us and frankly, we have no idea when we will be able to catch up with our mortgage payments," we'd admitted in defeat, planning to hand over the deed. Instead, the owners were friendly, sympathetic, upbeat and encouraging. "You guys are doing a great job. No one else could do better. Keep doing what you're doing, and when the economy comes around, we'll sit together and figure out a way to restructure the debt." Good news. This was patient money. And obviously they knew there were no buyers out there for the land.

Another two years went by. We continued to work on the project, paid our direct bills through escrow, and instead of taking any money for ourselves, we made sure that our contractors and suppliers were all paid up. We were working hard and making progress.

By 1968 there was a glimmer of activity in the Tucson market. But just as the cycle began to turn, out of the blue we received a lawyer's letter telling us that we were almost $400,000 in default, that we had 60 days to bring the mortgage current or the owners were going to take our land and the water company. We felt bitterly deceived. I had about 200 water customers, and I estimated that the company would be worth $2 million to $3 million one day. Now, just as the economy was allowing us to imagine a reasonable success, our "friends" in Detroit wanted to seize everything and sell it to another builder. We'd been betrayed.

I called my lawyer in a fury. "Can they do this?" He assured me that they did indeed have the right, and that my only out was to declare Chapter 11 bankruptcy and ask the court for time to reorganize. My blood was boiling. Worse, I could ask for a Chapter 11 only if we had unpaid bills to contractors, suppliers, professionals or other unsecured creditors. Being the upstanding local guys that we were, we kept current with our suppliers and other than to the mortgage holders on the land, we owed money to no one but the bank—and that was secured by the developed lots. But somehow, with the cooperation of about 10 contractors, we came up with a set of bills that amounted to about $30,000 in unsecured debts that the bankruptcy court could recognize and grant us the Chapter 11 to "protect." It was a pittance, but it was enough.

The court gave us two years to restructure, but we were in and out of bankruptcy in nine months. At that time it was the largest successful Chapter 11 bankruptcy in Tucson's history.

Every one of the contractors got paid, the lenders got their money and our homeowners got their homes. But I never forgot what it felt like to be double-crossed and betrayed.

Not the number you want to hear

The anger and stress were battering my body. Every six months I'd be back at the hospital for this test or that, and in the midst of the bankruptcy, just as my 40th birthday was nearing, I must've looked like a prime candidate for a meltdown. My doctor asked me if I'd be willing to participate in a new study that would compare my biological age to my chronological age. He explained that I would be part of a national research study on adults aged 25 to 75 to determine norms at different ages.

I was curious, so I went in for an afternoon of detailed medical testing and physiological measuring, which included going on a biofeedback machine to test my stress levels. When we were done, the doctor thanked me and said it would be about three weeks before he would get all the information back with an answer.

As I waited my anxiety kicked in. "I'm going to be 40, and suppose this thing comes back and says I'm 45 biologically," I thought. "Or, God forbid, maybe I'm 50 biologically." I wasn't optimistic. This had been the worst single year in my business life, and I couldn't think of a single reason I should be any luckier with my health.

As promised, about three weeks later the doctor called me back. My heart started racing when I heard his voice. "Mel, we've got some good news and some not so good news," he said.

Uh-oh.

"The good news is that we didn't find anything medically wrong with you that we didn't already know about."

I held my breath, waiting for the other shoe to drop and thinking, "Thank you very much! Of all my friends I'm the sickest guy in the crowd, but at least they didn't find anything new."

"But here's the not-so-good news," he continued.

Oh boy, I was thinking, here it comes.

"Actually," he said, "when we compared your results to the data bank norms you are living in the body of a 65- to 70-year-old man."

CHAPTER 5

Save My Life? Or Just Blow it Up?

———•◆•◆———

I can still remember which phone I was on when I got the news. Only a guy from New Jersey moves out to Tucson and builds the only house in town with a basement. It was 1,400 square feet with a wet bar, a pool table, ping-pong table and plenty of room to dance. But I never went down except to play pool or ping-pong, and that's what I was doing when I took Dr. McFadyen's call. I was braced for something bad. But this was something else. I held the receiver away from my ear as the words "body of a 70-year-old man" sank in. After a few seconds, the doctor said, "Mel, are you still there?"

"Yeah, doc. I'm here but I can't process what you just told me. I don't fully understand."

"It's important and worth talking about," he said. "Why don't you make an appointment when you have a chance and come in?"

When I had a chance? How about right now? If I could have been in his office in 10 minutes, I would have.

It took me three days to get in to see him, and by that time, I was a basket case. The first words out of my mouth when I sat down were, "Doc, did you give me a death sentence the other day? I'm thinking that if I'm in a 65- or 70-year-old body and I'm now 40, by the time I'm 50, some of my organs will be 80 or 85 years old and might decide they've had it. End of story."

I was more fearful at that moment than I had ever been in my life. Then the doctor said the magic words: "There are some things you can do about it..."

He said it almost casually, as if I might not be interested.

"OK," I said. "Tell me quick."

"The first thing is, you've got to lose 50 pounds."

Great. I'd never had any real success dieting or restricting my intake. I started gaining weight in my 20s and 30s. And for 10 years, Dr. McFadyen had been telling me: "You need to lose 20 pounds." Or 30. Or 40. And occasionally 50. I looked him straight in the eye and said, "Mac, since you've been treating me, honest, I think I've lost 1,000 pounds." That wasn't far from the truth. Later I calculated that it was really between 600 and 700 pounds that I'd lost yo-yoing during the last 10 years. Every time I went to him, four or five times a year, he would swivel around from his desk to a console piled high with papers and pull out the latest diet craze, inevitably a "deprivation" diet. Grapefruits, bananas, 1,000-calorie, protein, low-carb, all meat, no meat—I tried all of them. I'd go on the fad diet of the month, and as my weight would go south, so would my temperament. I would lose 15, 20, 25 pounds, but I'd be so impossible to live with that Enid would threaten to kick me out of the house.

So I'd go off the diet and back to doing everything I'd done before. And the next time I was in for a checkup, my weight would be up again, and I'd get another new super-effective weight loss plan. This pattern actually played out throughout my 30s and 40s. I'd shrink down to 185 and balloon up to 210 or 220. Ninety-five percent of the time, I weighed more than 195. I could lose weight in the short term, but no one in all those years had been able to tell me how to keep it off.

Now it was urgent. Fifty pounds. I was 210 again, eating my nightly ice cream, drinking too much alcohol, eating out too much. Getting to 160 wasn't achievable, 170 maybe. I had the fear of God in me. "All right," I told myself. "This time it's for real." Because if I didn't lose the weight, I'd be dead in 10 years.

There was something else, the doctor said. "You've got to exercise." Exercise wasn't in my repertoire, and it hadn't been since I was 8. Didn't he know that with my asthma, exercise could kill me? The thought of jogging in the predawn hours with my inhaler was ludicrous. And who had time for that? What was I supposed to do? Bike to Phoenix when it was

110 degrees? I gave McFadyen all my excuses. He said, "Try walking."

"When I walk I get cramps in my legs," I said. No can do.

The third thing he told me was that I needed to learn how to control stress. The biofeedback machine had shown that mine was off the charts.

"How do I do that?" I asked. This was 1968, and the worst year of my business life so far.

He had no techniques or strategies to offer, just one bit of advice: "Mel," he said, "You have to learn how to take things less seriously."

Get thee to a fat farm

I didn't say a word about any of this to Enid for quite a few days. She'd asked me why the doctor was calling, but I'd made something up, and I didn't mention my visit to his office. I was too shaken. When I finally told her what was going on, she was adamant: "Get yourself in a program, go to a fat farm and get yourself on a diet you can stick to!" I might have laughed it off before—a fat farm! But I knew I had to find a way to turn my health around, and I thought the idea was brilliant. I didn't want to go on another stupid diet that wouldn't work. Maybe I could go away and learn something. We found a place in Mexico called Rancho La Puerta that seemed like a good bet. It had a good reputation—vegetarian diet, even a fitness program, something new in those days.

I went with the idea that I would stay for two weeks, lose some weight and give good health a kick-start. I'd pay attention to my diet, get a little exercise. A couple of weeks of that and I felt sure that I could turn back my biological clock. I was scared enough to hand over control of my business to my partner for the first time in as long as I could remember. I hadn't had a vacation in ages. But I was desperate.

A quick glance around told me I was the only guy at the resort. I was intimidated. I thought I'd start out slowly, with a stretch class. So on my first morning, I tucked myself into the very back of the room and waited as people filed in. One by one they sat down cross-legged on the floor, and at 9 sharp, the instructor came dancing into the room, singing, "Good morning, ladies!" Then she spotted me crouched against the wall. "Oh! Welcome, sir!" she said cheerfully. Every head turned to look at me. "Why don't you come up to the front of the room so you can see better!"

Why not? Because I'd rather die.

"OK! What we're going to do is sit with our backs at right angles and our legs flat out on the floor."

Ha. With my legs straight out in front of me, I'm prone.

"And you sir, in the back? There are some pillows up against that back wall you can use to prop your butt up."

Turning back to the class, she said, "Now we're going to gradually bend forward. Just bend forward, and do whatever's comfortable for you. Don't overstrain or overstretch."

For me, the whole thing was a stretch and a strain. Women are just hinged differently from guys. Regardless of size or age, everyone in front of me was able to grab her ankles. Many of the women had their hands locked around the soles of their feet, and a few of the yoga types were folded flat at the waist, with their breasts pressing down on their quads, fingertips beyond their feet. I could barely reach my knees.

Sweating, with my knees up under my chin, I was straining and reaching, trying to mimic what the women were doing with such ease. My face was bright red. It may have been the most embarrassing moment of my life. Was everybody looking at me? Was anybody? No. They were all completely absorbed in their own efforts. But I felt so humiliated I refused to go into another class. "I'll just walk by myself. I'll sit around the pool and read," I thought. Maybe I'd lose weight on the diet, and maybe I'd even be able to figure out how to walk without getting cramps in my legs. That would be enough.

No one on the staff paid any attention to me, but the guests were very friendly. They'd motion me over to sit with them at the table in the dining room, or come upon me as I was reading by the pool. "Come on, Mel! Join us!" I tried, but it was all recipes and cooking and who'd had twins recently, and which one had had a Cesarean. I'm not shy, and I can hold my own in a conversation, but here I was completely out of my element.

It was raining on the third morning of my stay, so I sat in the lobby with my book. A woman was checking out, and I overheard her say that she was driving back to Del Mar, Calif. That meant she had to drive right past the San Diego airport! I approached her at the desk. "Would you give me 15 minutes to put my bags together?" I asked. "And drop me off at the airport?"

She said fine. And so, on Day Three of my healthy resolve, I hitchhiked out of the fat farm and went home. I hadn't lost a pound.

Enid was angry with me when I got back, but I didn't want to talk about it. I dealt with this setback the way I dealt with everything else. I buried myself in denial, ice cream and work.

Back to work

The business was still in crisis. After the bankruptcy, I was back to square one, so I tried working for someone else. It made me one miserable guy. I did learn something useful in the process, though: I couldn't stand not being the one who made the decisions, and when I tried, it was tough for me to get in my car and go home and be nice. I left the job in six months and went back to working for myself, on my own land.

As part of the Chapter 11, to settle the bank debt, I had sold about a third of the 400 acres I'd bought for Sabino Vista. But since everyone in town knew that I had made good on my obligations even in the darkest times, the banks had faith in me. So, when the market began improving, I was able to borrow enough money to buy more land to develop. In the '70s, I started building homes again.

I had several new subdivisions, and as a builder I was moving up the food chain, building on larger lots, one-acre lots, with houses that sold for $40,000 to $60,000. My local bank gave me mortgage commitments for a new subdivision and I was on top of the world, confident that at least financially, the dark days were behind me.

But at home, things had long been imploding. The ups and downs of our life had twisted my relationship with Enid. She had turned inward, and I had become a screamer and an arguer. I was convinced I had reasonable points of view, but unlike the guys I bossed around on construction sites, she wouldn't listen. Worse, when I started to argue, she would just turn her back and walk away. And that would infuriate me even more.

During all those years, she took care of our kids, our house, our parents (who had moved to Tucson) and kept up our social life, and in my unenlightened eyes, she was just doing her job—women's work, I thought. My job as a man was to provide for my family and figure out how to stay in the game when circumstances put me on the defensive. We didn't have a clue how to communicate with each other.

Meltdown

Each of us was awash in unmet needs, and we were headed for a train wreck. Enid began looking elsewhere for warmth. She was distant, and I was lonely. I discovered that there were a lot of women who were willing and available. Not that I was consciously looking, but you can get pretty close to a woman when you are building her home. I was in my early 40s, and I'd assumed that a much younger woman wouldn't give me a second look. I couldn't believe how many women found me "charming." I had a series of short-term affairs in 1970-71, a longer one in '72, and in August 1972, I moved out of our house and into an apartment.

For the next several months, I bounced between places. Enid and I would reconcile and I'd come home, determined to try again, but I'd never stay long. The last affair had turned serious, and I was torn between two women. It was a classic, stupid, midlife crisis.

Our separation turned into a formal divorce in June 1973, and in July, Enid left Tucson and moved back to New Jersey with our dogs, the housekeeper, a parakeet and Amy, who was 14 and in middle school. Jay was 18, leaving for college in California and determined to remove himself from the whole drama.

My life was out of control, and work was no refuge. In fact, in short order it was just another crisis to add to the heap. That

July the government raised interest rates, and mortgage rates skyrocketed. Many of my customers had bought homes based on being able to afford a monthly payment tied to a lower interest rate, and when my bank reneged on its commitments and demanded the higher rate, I was forced to sue.

Another catastrophe. I couldn't move my lots because with interest rates so high, mortgages were out of reach. I could barely afford the payments on my own construction and land loans. Once again, I was in financial trouble. I was also seriously depressed, with my weight ballooning, my health in jeopardy and my marriage and family in shreds.

In the months the suit moved through the courts, we were in limbo. Ultimately I won—in 1974, the court made the bank honor its mortgage commitment for the houses that I had already built and sold. But there was a catch. It wasn't required to offer the original lower rates for any of my unsold properties. Fortunately, I quickly found a new savings and loan that wanted my business, and I again could provide affordable mortgages.

In the midst of all this, temporary insanity took over completely. I'd gotten involved with a young woman when I was building a house for her and her husband in early 1972. She was 25. Short shorts, long legs—very sexy, and young enough to be my daughter. And she was obviously attracted to me. I couldn't believe that she was interested—I was 44. We began what started out, for both of us, as a casual affair.

But things intensified fast when she told her husband about the affair, naively thinking a liberated guy like him wouldn't mind. He was liberated all right. He liberated himself from their marriage the day she told him and left her with their two kids. I felt responsible, and that guilt was a major factor in my divorce and Enid's leaving.

On Labor Day weekend, after Enid and Amy had moved to New Jersey, I invited the young woman on a trip with a couple of friends from Tucson to a resort in San Diego. My friend Ken had a yacht in the marina, and the four of us went out for a day's expedition, a few miles off the coast of Mexico, lounging on the deck with icy drinks. As a joke, my buddy's young wife said, "Hey, we're out in international waters and Ken's the captain! I bet he could marry you! Can't the captain of a boat marry people?"

We all thought this was riotously funny. So, as my girlfriend and I stood side by side in our bathing suits, the "captain" intoned, "Do you take this woman to be your lawful wedded wife?" I said, "I do," but in my head I was saying, "I don't." (After all, this was only in fun.) And then we dived into the ocean.

Then our friends said, "Wouldn't it be something if the wedding was legal!" I pooh-poohed the idea that the mock wedding could be legally binding. It was a joke, for God's sake! But as I put down the legality of the ceremony, my girlfriend became increasingly angry, insulted that I didn't take her seriously as a potential wife. From her perspective she had a lot on the line. I hadn't had any intention of marrying her, but this is where my temporary insanity became full blown irrationality.

When we got back to port, we went out for drinks, and there behind the bar was a grizzled old sea captain. Great! We'd ask him if our "marriage" was legal. When he shook his head, signifying "absolutely not," I laughed. My girlfriend didn't even crack a smile.

She was seething. At dinner the next night, she was still so furious that she left the restaurant and started walking down the dark highway. What was I supposed to do? Let her leave me too? Just like Enid? I called the airline and got us tickets to Las Vegas for the next morning. We flew in at 9 a.m. and were back in San Diego by noon—married. For real. And it was all too clear that I'd made a big mistake.

When Enid heard that I'd gotten married only six weeks after she'd moved to New Jersey, she wouldn't talk to me, and we communicated only through our daughter. I tried to make my peace with what I'd done, but I was lonely. It was one thing to be a single guy dating around Tucson, and quite another to try to adjust to life as a newly married man, with a new family that included two small children. I missed Amy desperately, and to be quite candid, I missed Enid and felt lost without her. I was in a low mood when we went to my new father-in-law's house for Thanksgiving. And when my new wife asked what was wrong, I answered, "I miss my family. This is my first Thanksgiving without my family." She was sharp. "We're your family now," she said quickly. But, in my heart, I knew that wasn't true.

The following week, I was hospitalized with a hiatal hernia attack, and although my new wife came morning and evening to visit, I had a lot of time alone to think. Every day I'd ask myself, "How do I get out of this?" I called Enid from the hospital, and I was relieved when she came to the phone. "All I can think about is you," I told her. Enid's tone was curt. "Well, you're married to someone else now. There's not much I can do about that."

I was desperate to find a way out. The week after I got home from the hospital we had an argument. On the way home from a basketball game, I offhandedly announced that my doctor had told me I needed to drop a lot of weight quickly or risk serious health consequences. It was true. I had decided to take myself to a fat farm.

"You're not going without me!" she said.

"Yes, I am," I replied. "You need to spend time with your kids. They've been through a lot in the last year. I'm going by myself."

We fought all the way home, and when we got there, she slammed the door in my face and locked it. I had the key in my hand but I didn't use it. I knew it was my moment, and I was grateful. I drove to my office and slept on the couch.

"The whole thing is wrong," I said when I called her in the morning. "Wrong for me. Wrong for you. You need to go live your life, and so do I." I arranged a time when she would be out of the house so I could remove my clothes and belongings, and I moved into a bedroom at my mother's house. A few months later the divorce was final. We'd been married just three months. It was an expensive mistake.

How had this happened? Why had I felt the need to fly to Las Vegas for a quickie wedding in the first place? I think now that the jolt of breaking up her marriage had left me feeling unbearably guilty. And the thought of going home to an empty house if she walked out in anger was even worse. I was terrified of being alone. With Enid no longer my rock, my anchor, I felt like I was lost at sea.

Thousands of miles away, I knew she was thriving. Reconnecting with old friends, dating, entertaining family, both hers and mine. She was making a new life without me. But I held out hope that she'd take me back. In fact, I'd spent the month before I separated from my new wife testing the waters. Enid had been in Yuma for her nephew's bar mitzvah in November, and my parents, who continued to adore her, had been invited. A few days after the party, my father came into my office on a mission. "I want you to know that Enid misses you," he said.

"She won't even talk to me," I said, dejected.

"Mel, she still cares," he said.

I wrote to her right away, and I was shocked that she wrote back. Enid remembers that I had called her crying, saying I was miserable and lonely in the new relationship. She told me frankly that she "loved it" that I was unhappy, but unfortunately she had to get ready for a date that night and couldn't talk at length. Soon we were writing letters back and forth. She sent them to my post office box, and for that brief stretch before my divorce, it was as though the woman I'd been married to for so many years had become the other woman.

Jay's school in California was a short flight from Tucson, and we managed to see each other reasonably frequently. But Amy was 2,500 miles away with her mother in New Jersey, and I missed her fiercely. So I asked her to spend Christmas vacation with me in Tucson, and with Enid's permission she came. I wrapped my arms around her when she got off the plane, enormously grateful. At that moment I understood just how much I loved and missed my family, and how desperate I was to get Enid to come back to me.

When I asked Enid what she wanted for her birthday in January 1974, her answer thrilled me. "You," she said.

"Would it be OK if I flew out there to celebrate?" I asked.

I made my reservations instantly. This was a thaw if ever I'd heard one. By coincidence, Enid was hosting a party for the cousins on my side of the family on the same weekend, and she said she was going to tease them by introducing her "new" boyfriend who "looked a lot like Mel."

I had boarded the plane in Tucson, drove from JFK in a snowstorm and got lost trying to find the address of the house where she was living. But nine hours later, I was at her doorstep. I rang the bell, opened the door and walked in. "Oh my God!" one of my cousins said. "He does look a lot like Mel!" Another cousin fainted. After lots of hugs, I started to make a tour around the house Enid had purchased.

"How could you buy a place like this?" I asked. "You knew I was coming back for you."

Enid remembers that even though she had moved across the country, burned our wedding albums, melted down her wedding ring into a teardrop and divorced me, she had to admit that we weren't done yet. The energy and love between us were still there. But first, I had to win back her trust.

I began flying East every third weekend, and returning to Tucson for the workweek, courting her. This time, I knew how important it was to nurture my wife. By summer, I had persuaded her to move back to Tucson so that Amy could start the school year and we could be together, living in our own house. We lived "in sin" until Nov. 16, 1974. That day, on the 22nd anniversary of our very first date, we got married for the second time. Enid likes to refer to herself as my third wife. She thinks it makes her sound younger. I refer to her as my true love and my soul mate. For that's what she is.

A seed is planted

The Zuckerman family had weathered the great crisis of our divorce, and both of us were working harder at communicating. One evening in 1975, while I was in one of my moods over some business crisis or other, Enid took a long hard look at me, almost clinically assessing my anxiety-rich life as a developer. She fixed me with her give-me-no-bull stare and said, "Is this really what you want to do for the rest of your life?"

It was a prophetic and important question, and it registered with me. I answered her honestly. "No, I don't. But what else is there for me to do? I've got to earn a living, and I won't go back to being an accountant."

She thought for a minute, and said quietly, "Why don't we open a fat farm in Tucson?"

I laughed her off. A dumb idea. A ridiculous idea!

Enid was wiser than I. She was already exercising and eating with care. She reasoned that people were "going to get the idea sooner or later that they have to exercise, eat nutritiously and keep their weight under control if they want to stay healthy."

It went in one ear and out the other, but that ridiculous idea somehow stuck in the back of my mind.

CHAPTER 6

The Aha! Moment

W ith Enid and Amy back in our house, I felt like a changed man. Business was rebounding too. I may have taken a beating from the economy, but my reputation was unscathed, and the next few years were excellent. I was president of the home builders' association, and when IBM moved to Tucson, I went over to give a talk. All the engineers wanted me to build their homes.

1976 and 1977 were the two best years I ever had as a developer. I was able to pay off all my land loans, and even build a substantial nest egg. By 1978, I was the only small home builder in Tucson who had survived the perils of the last two decades. I'd built 1,200 homes and more than 400 apartments. Professionally, I felt pretty good about myself.

But I was still that middle-aged guy in the body of a

70-year-old, now much the worse for wear. Mortality was knocking again, and this time I could hear it.

"If only..."

A moment that changed everything for me came in 1977, when my father died of cancer. Norman Zuckerman, whom I'd revered and loved, had been a steady two- to three-pack-a-day smoker for most of his adult life, and by the time he was 76, the habit had caught up with him. He didn't feel well, and since he hadn't been to a doctor in more than five years, my mother and I talked him into going in for a checkup.

The doctor called soon after to ask if Enid and I would come into the office to be with my mom and dad when he delivered the test results. "The news," he told us, "will not be good."

The four of us went in and waited anxiously in our chairs. "Mr. Zuckerman," the doctor told my dad, "you have inoperable lung cancer, and I can't hold out much hope."

Dead quiet in the room.

"How long?" my father asked (or maybe that was me).

"Not long. Months, not years."

My father turned ashen. I saw a slight tremble in his hand. He stood up and reached into his pocket for his pack of Camels. I half expected him to tap one out of the bottom and light it up as he had done thousands of times in my life when he was nervous. Instead he crushed it between his hands and threw it on the edge of the doctor's desk.

"I'll quit!" he said. "This time I mean it! I will quit!" True to his word, he never smoked another cigarette.

Norman Zuckerman was a changed man. But his resolve came far too late. He passed away six and a half months later, one month after his 77th birthday. His self-recriminations were constant during those last six months. I can still hear him saying, "If only…" "If only I had quit smoking sooner … If only…" In those final weeks, my father used the phrase, "If only I had…" more than any other words. "If only…" meaning, "I wish I had done it differently. I wish I had stopped that time. Remember all those times I tried? If only I had. …" I was his only child, his only son, and every day he would come to my office and ask, "Mel, how long do you think I have?"

I realized that my father's whole life was full of regret. The process of his dying was excruciating to watch as his body failed and he struggled to breathe. I mourned for the good and gentle man who had been the emotional pillar of my life as a child and had continued to be a supportive presence throughout my adult life. I mourned for myself a little as well. Just shy of 50—a milestone birthday for any man—I had to acknowledge in my own dim, unconscious way that I too was in danger of being the kind of man whose dying words might be, "If only…" How many diets had I started? How many times had I tried to change? At some deep level, I was planting the seed for a life without regret. I resolved to lose some weight and get myself fit. I was still asthmatic, overweight and out of shape. In a kind of despair about my own health. But this time I was ready to save my life.

Aha! at the Oaks

I was determined to make the so-called second half of my life much different from the first. My simple goal was to lose 30 pounds before my 50th birthday in May. I'd go back to Rancho La Puerta, and this time I would stay. No hitchhiking out, no skulking away from exercise class. I'd lose weight and work on getting in shape. Enid called to book me a room, but they were full, with a long waiting list. I didn't want to wait.

Then, browsing through magazines, we found a small advertisement for a spa in Ojai, California The ad showed a pretty woman in a leotard standing next to a swimming pool, holding a polka-dotted ball over her head. A bunch of women in the swimming pool, also holding polka-dotted balls, were smiling for the camera. The ad read "Lose a Pound a Day with Sheila!"

"Sheila" was Sheila Cluff, the owner of the Oaks at Ojai. I looked at Enid, she looked at me, and I said, "Eh? Maybe I should try it."

This time I drove my own car, just to be sure that I could get out if I wanted out. I had no idea where Ojai was, and of course, since I'm not the sort of man who asks directions, what should have been a nine-hour drive took me 13. Enid rode along with me—I think she wanted to make sure that I actually checked in at the spa.

We both assumed that the best outcome was that I'd lose 10 pounds. Maybe 15. And I would come home with a looser belt. I planned to stay only as long as it took to reach that modest goal. Ten days. Maybe two weeks.

The basic premise at the Oaks was simple: Give the guests a calorie-restricted diet, a lot of exercise and a massage at the end of the day. It was a proven recipe for success for the many guests—almost all women—who came and went, losing weight, going home thinner and coming back the next year to take off the same five or 10 pounds. Right after check-in, there was an orientation session for all of us new arrivals, where we gathered around the fireplace in the living room, finding chairs for the chat. As the only man among a dozen or so women, I stuck out, and I was more than a little worried that I was in for a replay of my earlier spa experience at Rancho La Puerta.

But there was something different about this place. Leading the session was one of the most remarkable women I have ever met, a tall, honey-haired pillar of confidence and vitality. That was Karma Kientzler, the fitness director at the Oaks. During the orientation, she had directed most of her eye contact at Enid, assuming that Enid was the guest, and I'd be leaving. So when the session ended, Enid went up to clarify things. "Hey, I'm not the one staying—he is," she told Karma. "And it's your job to keep him here."

Karma made a beeline for me. "Got a few minutes?" she said. "I'd really like to talk to you."

I was almost inarticulate. "Yeah. Sure."

"I'd really like to find out why you're here, and what you're hoping to accomplish during your stay."

"Why me?" I wondered as Karma stepped closer into my comfort zone.

She told me she'd picked up from my body language that part of me wanted to be there, and part of me wanted to be any place but at a fat farm. She said she'd decided to adopt me as her pet project. I was taken aback by her directness—I'd been on the premises all of an hour. By the time our short exchange was over, Karma had challenged every one of the myths I held about myself, and what I could or couldn't accomplish physically. Before I could come up with a good excuse for bailing out on the first activity of the day, Karma swiftly made arrangements for another instructor to lead the 7 a.m. walk for the other guests so she could walk with me alone. Who was this wild woman? Enid and I were agog. I imagined Enid smiling in amazement on her way to the airport.

The power of Karma

Bright and early the next morning, Karma collected me for my private morning walk, the brisk and traditional start to a day of fitness at the Oaks.

"How far are we going?" I asked her.

"A mile."

"I can't walk a mile," I said. "I've never been able to walk a mile. Didn't you hear me that I have a bad case of asthma? If I exercise too much, I'll get sick!" I whined, repeating the story I'd been telling since I was a wheezing 8-year-old.

Karma wasn't buying it. "We'll just walk at your pace."

And for the next half hour, we did, with Karma offering up a "can-do" to match every one of my "I can't's."

"We'll walk a mile."

"I can't walk a mile."

"Yes, you can."

Then she said, "We'll try to jog for 25 yards."

"I can't jog," I insisted.

"We'll go back to a walk as soon as you feel discomfort," she said.

"How fast will I have to walk?"

"As fast as is comfortable for you."

She was unflappable. Every time I said "I can't do that," she said, "I guarantee you, you can, and it will happen sooner and faster than you even think it is possible." That first day, it took 25 minutes for us to walk our mile. Karma was undeterred. "Good start," she said briskly, putting her stopwatch back in her pocket. "Now, we're going to be working out together twice a day, and I'll be phoning your doctor. I want to ask him about changing how you're medicating yourself for the asthma. If you changed the time of day you take your medicine, you might be able to manage exercise more easily. Oh, and by the way, we'll be working on breathing exercises. And some stretching exercises."

Again, I wondered: "Who is this woman?" But I already knew that resistance was futile. She and my doctor worked out a new schedule for my medication, agreeing that it would make it much easier for me to exercise in the morning. She began collecting me twice a day, and the two of us would walk and jog, and walk and jog, and jog and walk. Every day we'd jog a little longer than we'd walk.

On the 10th day, Karma pulled out her stopwatch again. We had jogged a mile and a half in 11 minutes and 38 seconds, or slightly better than an eight-minute mile. I'd chopped 17 minutes off my time from our first walk/run. Karma pulled a well-thumbed book from her satchel, a volume about aerobics written by the world famous Dr. Kenneth Cooper of the Cooper Clinic in Dallas. She quickly flipped it open. I was about to meet the numbers that would change my self-image for the rest of my life.

The chart she showed me tracked how quickly you should be able to traverse a mile and a half depending on your age. You could rate your fitness by comparing yourself to the rest of your age group. For example, if it took you 30 minutes to go a mile and a half at age 50, it meant you scored in the bottom 5% of your age group. On my first outing with Karma, it had taken me 25 minutes to go a mile; that translates as 37.5 minutes for a mile and a half, placing me perhaps at the bottom 2% of my age group. My first, baseline score wasn't one to instill any pride. But just a week and a half later I was jogging the equivalent of less than an eight-minute mile (a mile and a half in 12 minutes or less)! The chart showed that I'd zoomed from the bottom 2% to the top 5% in my age group! In 10 measly days!

Talk about a sense of empowerment! The top 5% in my age group? From the kid who couldn't run from home plate to first base or play singles tennis? I was euphoric.

After that wonderful, life-changing, morning run, I went to fitness classes at 9 and 10, and then I took a walk before lunch. Before I knew it, I was out the doors of the resort and walking down the main street of Ojai. Suddenly I was skipping, bouncing up and down like a grade school kid, high as a kite. All the little shops had awning signs in front that stuck out over the sidewalk, each about eight feet off the ground. With each skip I'd jump up and swat a sign. Then I'd click my heels. It had to be an odd sight, this fat guy in a T-shirt and shorts, clicking his heels. The shop owners and passersby were staring. But that day, I knew I was hooked for life. There was no way to turn back. I said out loud, "I want to feel this way forever!"

A moment to last a lifetime

Nothing in the previous 49 years, 10 months and some odd days of my life could've set me up to imagine I could achieve the joy of physicality that I had just experienced. Karma was my witness, my guide and my drill sergeant—my salvation.

I called Enid. "Something amazing is happening here," I told her.

"That amazing thing had better not be Sheila!" she said after a pause.

I assured her it was not Sheila and explained that I'd already lost 13 pounds, but another miracle was unfolding. "I don't know where this is going, but I want to give it a chance to play out because something life-changing is happening to me. And I think I should stay and see where this goes."

I wound up spending four weeks at Ojai and losing a total of 29 pounds. By the end of my stay, I was jogging three miles every single day. But it wasn't just my body that had changed. My spirit was different too. The two things that I'd thought were true about myself—that my body was a curse, and that it would always fail me—were wrong. I had proved that. It was my Aha! Moment.

It was like a light bulb going off in my consciousness, a flash when I realized that my life could be better—and that I had the power to make lasting change. Having an Aha! Moment is both thrilling and terrifying, because at the end of it, you understand that the decision to change course is yours, and yours alone.

Before my Aha! Moment, I had always thought of "health" as something that happened to you. Like having blue eyes, or being tall or short, or good at numbers. Now I knew better.

The week before I came home, I asked Enid to fly up. I needed her to be my partner and help me sustain this healthy lifestyle once we were back in Tucson. We'd have to figure out how to cook, where I'd find a trainer, and how I could find support to continue on my path. She was thrilled.

But I had something more important to discuss with her: "Remember that crazy idea you had about opening a fat farm in Tucson?" I said. "We're going to do it."

CHAPTER 7

Fleshing Out the Fantasy

—◆—◆—◆—

We talked nonstop all the way home. We were going to build a fat farm in Tucson! But it wasn't going to be like anything we'd seen or heard about. We'd build a resort where people would come to exercise, lose weight and learn the tools for healthy living. It wouldn't be Spartan, though. We'd make it so gorgeous and so much fun that they'd still feel as if they were on vacation. And with the encouragement we'd provide, our guests would come away empowered, just the way I had at the Oaks. This place would be so much more than a spa or a weight-loss camp that we'd need a new name for it. "How about calling it a fitness resort!" I told Enid. After all, wasn't getting fit the Aha! that changed my life? Fitness resort. That seemed right. There was just one catch: Neither Enid nor I nor anyone else in the world had any idea what it would really take to create a fitness resort. We needed to invent a brand new framework.

We tossed the question back and forth. What would this "thing" look like? What would the experience be? "Let's face it," Enid and I agreed, "Ojai is kind of limited." The spa facilities consisted of a sauna for two and a coed Jacuzzi. There was one large gym and a swimming pool outside, but not much else. We thought we could do better. Enid put it succinctly: "Let's just build a beautiful, unpretentious place with lots of fun activities for the guests—lots of gyms, an indoor pool and an outdoor pool—so they can feel like they are enjoying themselves while doing all the right things for their bodies," she said.

I agreed. The new resort also needed facilities like racquetball and tennis courts. It had to be male-friendly. I wanted it to be a place where guys with weight issues, the ones who were stressed out and needed to get on an exercise program, could feel at home. I wanted a place for guys like me.

"We should build the kind of resort where we'd be comfortable, where we would choose to go on vacation," Enid said. That approach had worked for us in the home-building business, and it seemed natural to try it here. But we knew there was a lot more to creating our fantasy place than facilities. As we talked, we realized that even though Sheila, Karma and the staff at the Oaks had so little to work with, they'd still managed to give me an experience that changed my life. I wanted to somehow pass along my Aha! Moment. That was my touchstone.

Hour after hour, as we headed south from Ojai, we dissected the concept. We grasped how desperate many people must be to lose weight if they were willing to put up with bare-bones fat farms. Those certainly weren't places that people would choose if they wanted to go on vacation and work on their health at the same time. The spas on the other end of the spectrum seemed to focus mostly on pampering. I'd read a little about a fancy place called La Costa. Supposedly, it had some workout facilities, with separate spa facilities for men and women. The write-ups never focused on weight loss or lifestyle change. It seemed that the "spa" was a nice amenity for resort guests who primarily came for golf and tennis. "Maybe we should go and check it out," Enid said.

A plan took shape. We'd make the rounds of spas, resorts and fat farms, and try to see if there were any ideas we could use. Was there anything close to our vision?

It was nightfall when we pulled into our driveway in Tucson. Did we even stop for gas? Our conversation had lasted 600 miles, and perhaps for the first time in our 25 years of married life (minus 17 months for my bad behavior), we agreed on virtually everything. We had a shared vision. Many of the core concepts of our dream resort had been articulated, scribbled down as we drove. Next day, I went to my office to catch up on all that I'd missed, and I basked in the glowing responses to my new svelte silhouette. I was on fire.

Making things personal

I was a changed man, and there was no way I was going back to my old half-gallon-of-ice-cream life. I was running miles every day, and working out with Enid at the gym she'd been going to for years. The owner was a gymnast, and his idea of fitness training was working out on rings and trapezes, and doing 50 push-ups and sit-ups at the end of each session. There wasn't much room for backsliding given Enid's level of personal discipline! But truly, I was never tempted to backslide. Enid decided to cook for me, and asked for recipes from the chefs at Ojai. Never a great cook, at first she thought she got the recipes wrong because the dishes were almost inedible. So she went back to the grocery store for ingredients and did it all over again. It turned out that the spa food was just plain terrible. That became one of the must-haves on the list for "our spa": healthy, low calorie food that was worth eating—guiltless gourmet.

Meanwhile, I'd started to plan a wind-down to my own day-to-day involvement in the real estate development company so I could devote time to my next set of projects. I suspected that my resort idea would claim a large portion of my time. Of course, I couldn't envision how it would swallow my entire life—both business and personal.

Over the next few months, we did our research, visiting virtually every spa that might have something to teach us. It was like "Goldilocks and the Three Bears." This one was too fancy, this one was too bare bones ... nothing was just right. We didn't find a single place, regardless of the price or amenities, where the staff was trying to motivate guests to change their lives for the long term. At every spa we saw, you'd get results to take home, but no guidance at all about making them last. Much as we hoped to be able to say, "Good! Let's model our resort on that," the place we envisioned didn't seem to exist.

Our list of things we didn't like was much longer than the list of things that we did, and partway through our research, Enid said, "Let's forget about all the others and just focus on creating an experience that will be fun, educational and life-changing for people like us." So that's what we did.

I knew that making a personal connection with the guest was key. I still thought about how marooned I'd felt when I showed up at Rancho La Puerta 10 years before in 1968. You had only to look at me to see that I was unhappy, overweight and out of shape, and you'd think someone might've asked me questions like, "Have you exercised before? Are you looking to get on an exercise program? What's your main goal? Is it just to lose weight?" Instead, I got the skimpiest of orientations: "Dinner is at such and such an hour" and "We have five levels of exercise classes tomorrow, blah, blah, blah ..."

Nobody had asked me a thing about myself—they just wanted to know if I wanted to book a massage. And when I said yes, the reply was a brusque: "OK, go into that room and get your massage schedule."

I'd walked over to a woman sitting in a small space with a calendar on the desk in front of her. "I'd like to get two or three massages in the next week and maybe you can get me one at 3 in the afternoon, one at 4 in the afternoon, one at 5 in the afternoon."

She'd looked up at me, looked down at her book, and said, "Let me tell you when you're going to get your massages. We have a 10 tomorrow morning, we have an 11 Wednesday morning and we have something at 1 in the afternoon on Friday." What she didn't say was, "I'm sorry, sir."

My time with Karma had shown me that to succeed in helping people make a substantive personal change, it was essential to believe that the staff cared about you. I wanted our fitness resort to be a place where we'd get to know our guests—their hopes and concerns and preferences—starting with the first telephone conversation about reservations. When someone arrived at our resort, the first question should be, "What do you hope to accomplish during your stay?"

Today it's standard for a spa or health destination to ask you about your goals, but 30 years ago, it was a pioneering concept. I wanted people to be as changed by their encounter with us as I'd been changed by Karma—and the only way to do it was by tailoring the experience to the person. That's how we came to develop prescriptive programming for each guest, based on his or her needs and goals.

Ambitious as our goals were, Enid and I pictured operating our resort as a sort of mom-and-pop business. We wouldn't make any real money, but we'd get by. I figured that with my real estate, cash in the bank and my water company, I had already made enough money for us to live well but modestly, as we always had. I'd had 20 years of stress, and I didn't want any more. We just wanted the second half of our lives to be healthy and fun. Opening a fitness resort of our own would keep us fit, active and involved. We'd take exercise classes, eat good food, get massages every day … what could be more fun than that? The resort would support a fantasy life that we wanted to create for ourselves. Maybe we'd even cover our living expenses if we got lucky.

A fixer-upper—with magic

I put out the word that I was in the market for some land I could develop as a resort, and just days later my real estate broker came to tell me about a ranch that was for sale. It had been on the market a long time, he said, and the owner was dying of lung cancer. "I think he's really motivated to sell," the broker told me.

"Really?" I said. "Where is it?"

"You know the Double U Dude Ranch?"

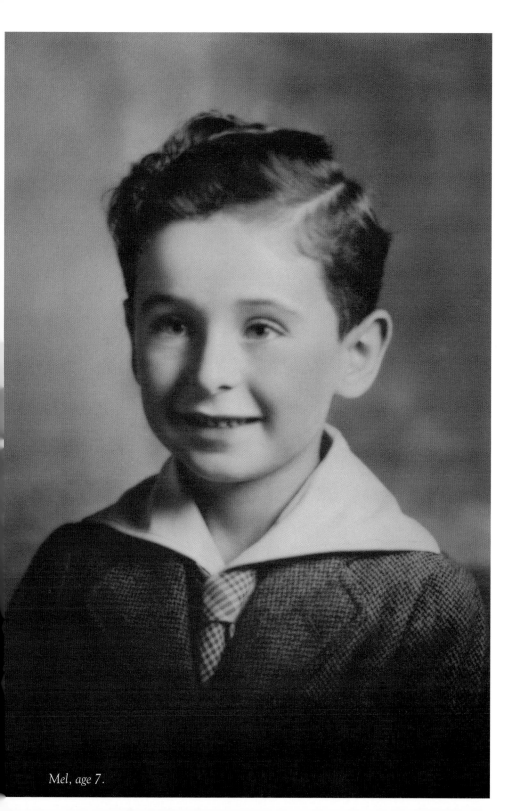

Mel, age 7.

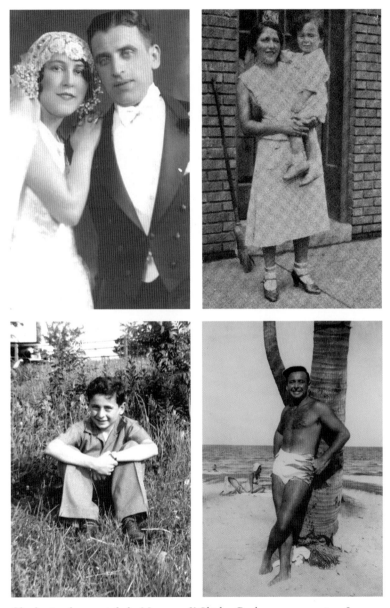

Clockwise from top left: Norman & Shirley Zuckerman marrying, June
12, 1927; Mom holding Mel, 1929 or 1930; Mel, 23, in Florida, 1951;
Mel at grandparents' farm, age 7 or 8.

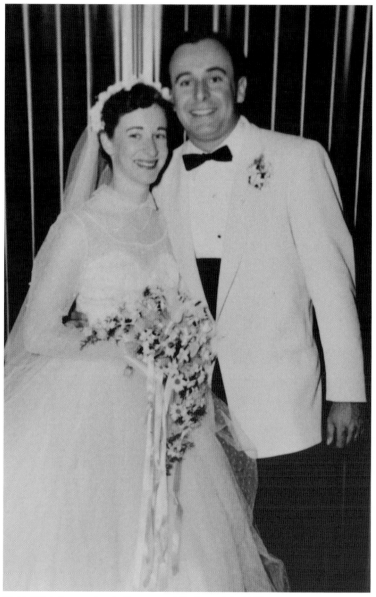

Enid & Mel marrying in Paterson, NJ, June 14, 1953.

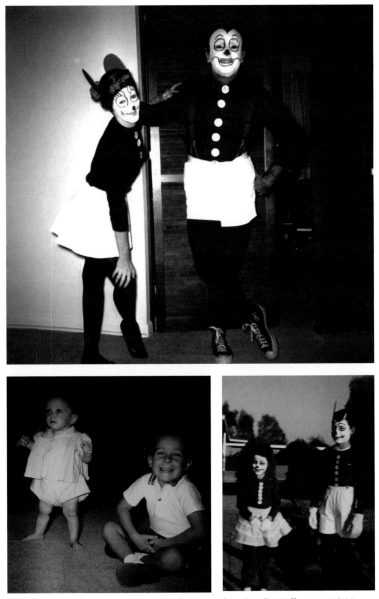

Clockwise from top: Minnie (Enid) & Mickey (Mel) Halloween 1964; Amy & Jay Halloween 1964; Amy, 2, & Jay, 5, 1960 or 1961.

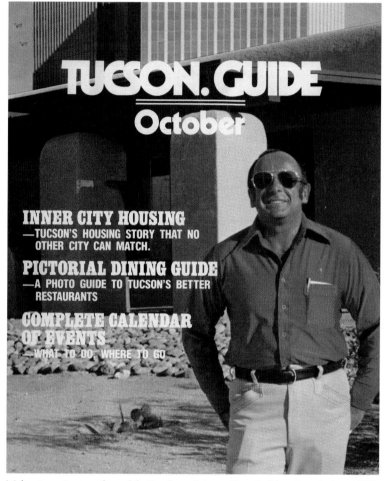

Mel as incoming president of the Southern Arizona Homebuilders Association, 1977.

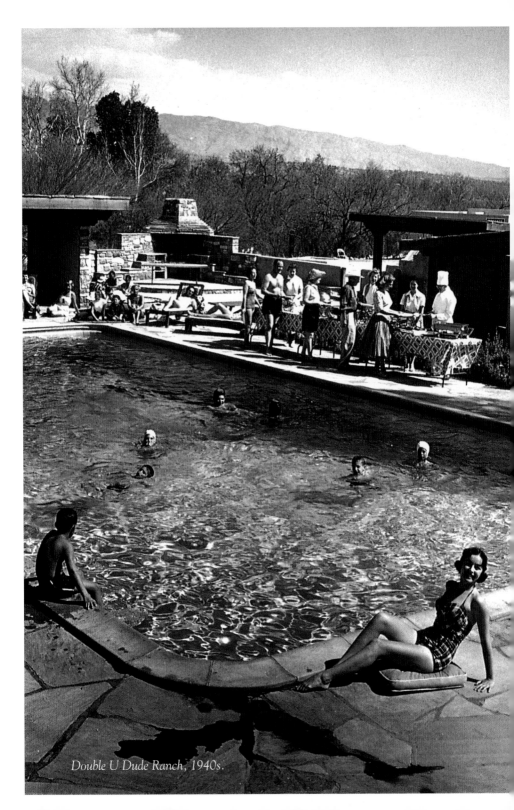

Double U Dude Ranch, 1940s.

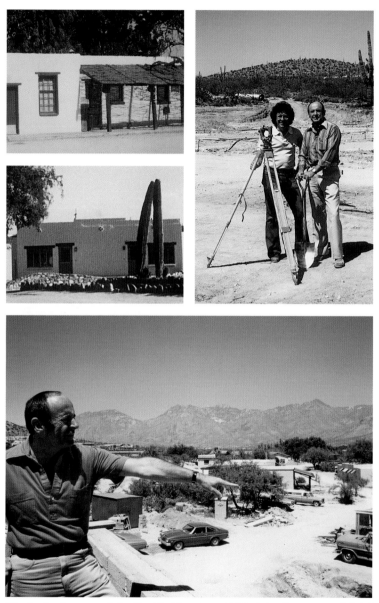

Clockwise from top left: *Double U casitas, 1978; John Campisano & Mel at groundbreaking, November 1978; Mel on the roof of the Spa building observing construction, 1979.*

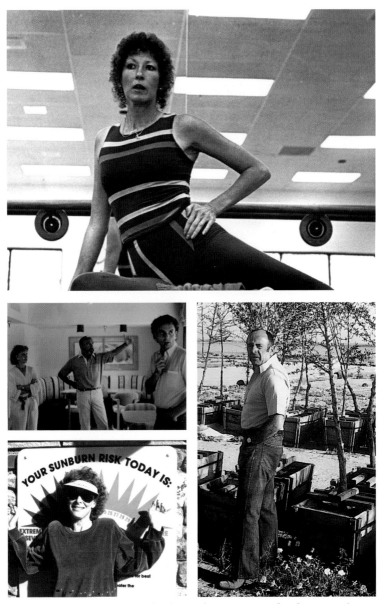

Clockwise from top: *Karma leading a class, 1980; Mel picking trees for landscaping Canyon Ranch in Tucson, 1979; Enid, 1981; Enid, Mel & Jerry during Dining Room remodel, circa 1986.*

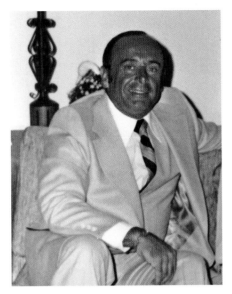

Mel Zuckerman,
age 49, June 1977.

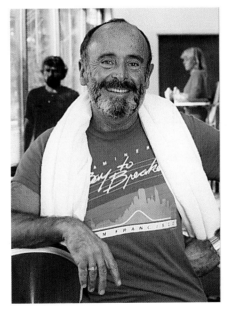

Mel Zuckerman, age 56,
June 1984, 30 pounds lighter
and decades younger.

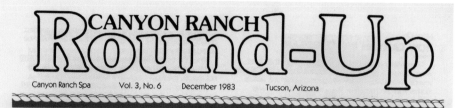

CANYON RANCH

Round-Up

Canyon Ranch Spa   Vol. 3, No. 6   December 1983   Tucson, Arizona

FOURTH ANNIVERSARY EDITION

Four years ago this month, Mel and Enid Zuckerman opened Canyon Ranch Spa, a resort dedicated to fitness, nutrition and overall well-being.

Today many of the people who helped form the original Canyon Ranch concept are still here, helping to improve and expand programs to better meet guest demands.

The fitness program is still headed by Karma Kientzler. The nutritious gourmet menus are still planned by Jeanne Jones and prepared by Peter Campbell. Deborah Morris continues to oversee herbal wraps, as well as giving wellness consultations. And Leah Kovitz continues to provide skin care services.

Other highly visible staffers who are part of the original team are Bernie Mayer, Chief of Security; John Knote, Front Desk Supervisor, and Phyllis Hochman, Trail Guide.

All around the ranch you'll find "original" staffers — teaching fitness classes, cooking meals, giving massages, attending in the locker rooms, tending the lush desert grounds or cleaning and maintaining everything.

These special staffers are responsible for the continuity of spirit at Canyon Ranch. Our thanks to all of them!

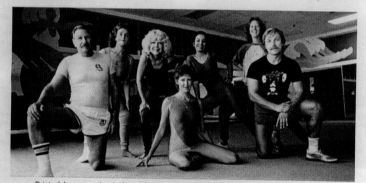

Original department heads: from left, Bernie, Phyllis, Jeanne, Karma, Leah, Deborah and Peter.

THE FOUNDATION OF CANYON RANCH IS LAID ON GOOD FRIENDSHIP

Actress June Lockhart settled eloquently back into her chair in the Canyon Ranch Cactus Room, thankful for the cushy comfort and the chance that evening to be inactive and nostalgic.

A certain softness in her eyes still gave her face that understanding quality familiar to millions of TV viewers as the pretty mother of Timmy on "Lassie" and of the galaxie-wandering family on "Lost in Space."

She is 57, but something about the determined glow of her skin and her persistent freshness made you know that she has paid a great deal of attention to her diet, her figure and her fitness in order to look and feel far younger than those years.

This particular night was a happy occassion for June, Canyon Ranch owner Mel Zuckerman and Executive Fitness Director Karma Kientzler — a reunion. The three first met five years ago at the Oaks, a spa in Ojai, Calif., where Karma was

general manager at the time.

Along with Karma, June was instrumental in changing Mel Zuckerman — from the overweight, exhausted, unhappy 50-year-old man he was when he came to the Oaks into the lean, happy, healthy, energetic, optimistic 55-year-old man he is today.

"You are indeed now all those things. Aren't you, Mel?"

"That's right, June."

So when Mel, Karma and June saw each other at Canyon Ranch recently to talk about rejuvenation, about health, determination, happiness and — most of all — their long friendship, their conversation was lively. It was sportive and bantering. It had the warm immediacy of old friends who once played pivotal roles in each others' lives and who are finally getting together after not seeing each other nearly enough.

(Continued p. 2)

Our newsletter for past guests, imaginatively called the Canyon Ranch Bi-Monthly Newsletter to begin with, soon became Round Up. *Several facelifts and another name change later, it's* Canyon Ranch Connection *today.*

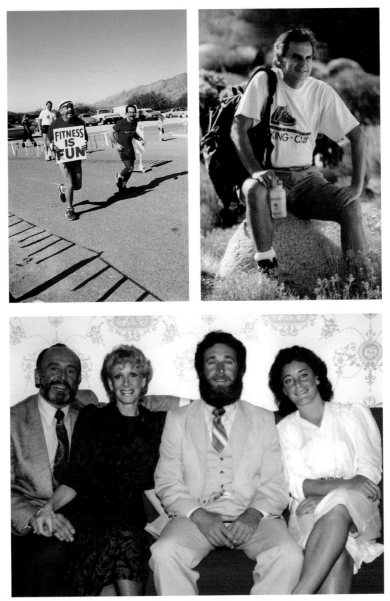

Clockwise from top left: Mel completing Canyon Ranch-sponsored marathon, 1982; Jerry Cohen on weekly hike with Mel, circa 1989; Mel, Enid, Jay and Amy, circa 1982.

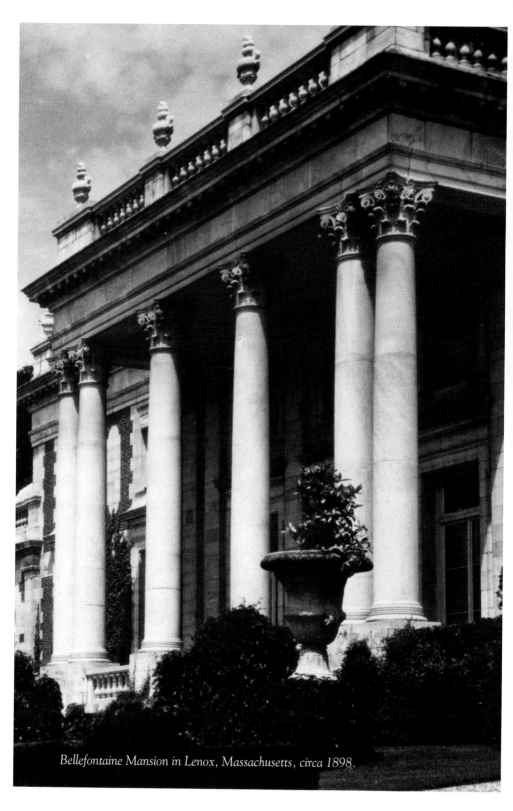

Bellefontaine Mansion in Lenox, Massachusetts, circa 1898.

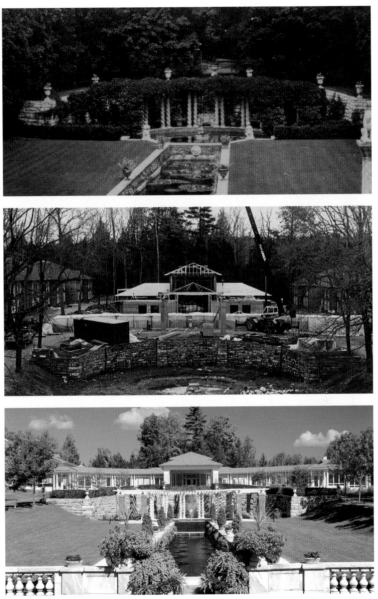

Top to bottom: *Bellefontaine Reflecting Pond, circa 1898; total reconstruction of the same area, 1989, new hotel and rooms in background; completed reconstruction, ready to open, September 1989.*

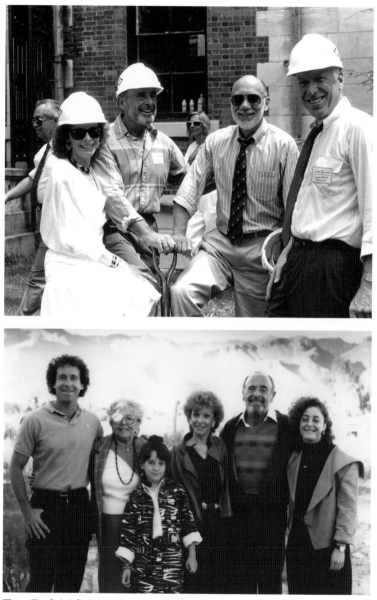

Top: *Enid, Mel, Bruce Berger, Dan Burack, at Lenox groundbreaking in August 1988.* **Bottom:** *Jay, Shirley, Nicole, Enid, Mel & Amy Zuckerman at the Health & Healing Center (Tucson) dedication, 1988.*

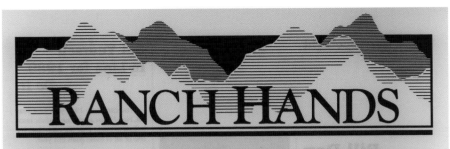

Health and Healing Center Dedication

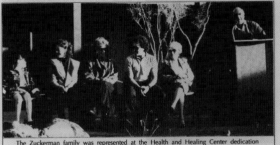

The Zuckerman family was represented at the Health and Healing Center dedication ceremony by (from left to right) Nicole, Amy, Enid, Jay, Mrs. Norman Zuckerman, and Mel.

The following excerpts are taken from the dedication speech given by Mel Zuckerman on December 20th for the new Health and Healing Center.

"And today, on its ninth birthday, Canyon Ranch is for the first time 'dedicating' some part of its facilities which are now the largest and most complete 'health, fitness and healing' facilities in the world. Enid and I have chosen to dedicate this Center because we believe that what goes on inside the walls of these buildings is what will lead Canyon Ranch into the 1990's and into the 21st century with a new vigor and expanded consciousness.

"It is very clear to me that though Enid and I passingly discussed the concept of owning a 'fat farm'/spa a couple of years earlier, that the deepening of that thought process never began until my experience in April 1978, a month before my 50th birthday—which would have never happened if my father hadn't

died in August of 1977. The passing of my Dad—to lung cancer caused by smoking—his very sad last months of life bemoaning his ill health and the knowledge of his impending death while recognizing that he had 'commissioned it,' and wishing he had lived his life differently and not smoked, was a powerful

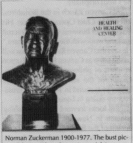

Norman Zuckerman 1900-1977. The bust pictured here and a plaque (text, right) are on display in the Health and Healing Center lobby.

lesson to me. Watching someone you love suffering not only their dying process, but mostly their past living process—I know was what planted, at that time, the unconscious 'seed' that grew into Canyon Ranch. I knew in the months following his death that I never wanted to have to look back as he did.

"Today, I'd like to honor the memory of my father, a man who in his death, it is my belief today, gave the world Canyon Ranch. The vision is ours—Enid's, and Jay's, and Jerry's, and Karma's and Dan's, and Phil's and dozens of others— but the impetus for the vision was Norman's—as it was he who planted its reason to be in my being—the powerful lesson to <u>never</u> look back with that depth of regret about how we live our lives.

"I'd like to now dedicate this Center to him and to that mission. The Health and Healing Center—a hub of love and knowledge—dedicated to a mission and a vision and to the memory of a very decent, caring and loving man."

Health and Healing Center

Dedicated December 1988

To the memory of Norman Zuckerman

a loving father and grandfather who in death, taught us the importance of making healthy choices so that we need never look back and wish we had lived our lives differently.

"If a man in the morning may hear the right way, he may die in the evening without regret." -Confucius

We hope this center helps you take responsibility for your own health and well-being.

The Zuckerman Family

Canyon Ranch Employee Newsletter

A dream come true – we announce the opening of the Health & Healing Center, dedicated to the memory of my father, in our staff newsletter.

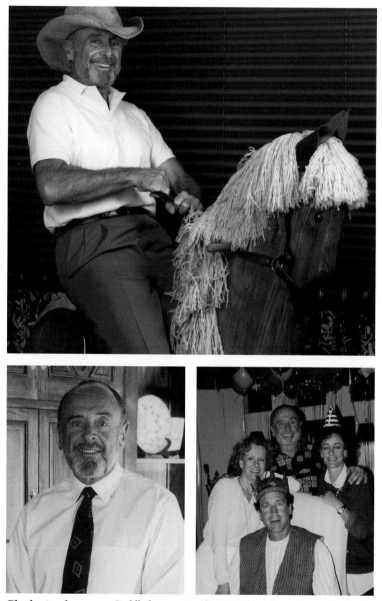

Clockwise from top: *Saddled up on Enid's 1988 birthday gift to Mel; Enid, Jay, Mel & Amy celebrating Jay's 40th birthday, May 1995; Mel, circa 1988.*

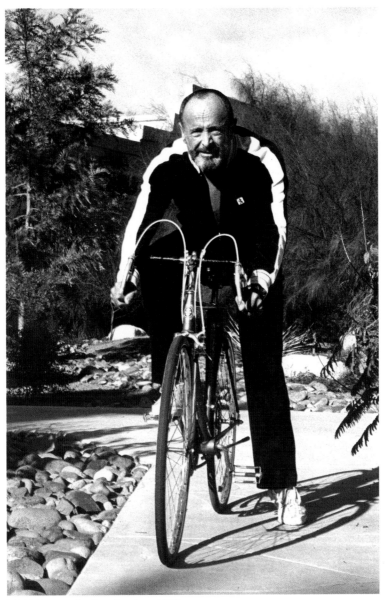

Mel biking at the Ranch, circa 1985.

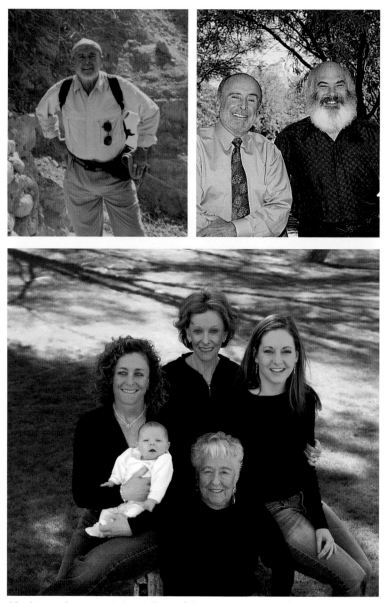

Clockwise from top left: *Mel on a hike, circa 2002; Mel & Andy Weil, circa 2001; four generations of Zuckerman women, 2004 – clockwise from left: Amy (holding Talia Rose), Enid, Nicole & Shirley.*

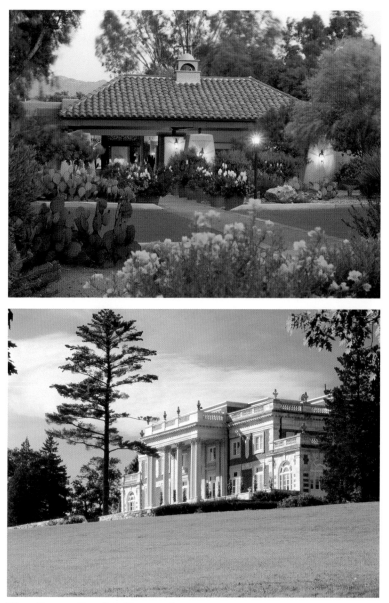

Top: *Canyon Ranch in Tucson, Arizona;*
Bottom: *Canyon Ranch in Lenox, Massachusetts*

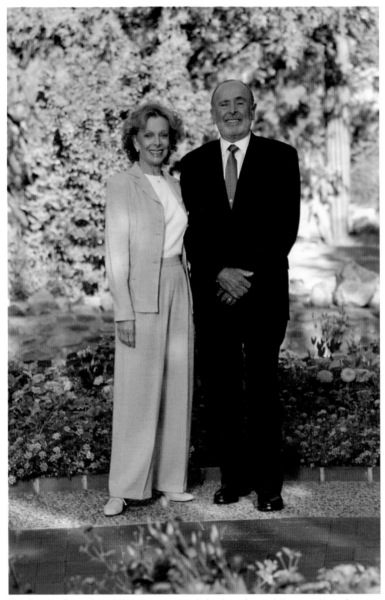

Enid & Mel on the 25th anniversary of the founding of Canyon Ranch.

"Wait a minute! I think I visited someone there 15 years ago. But I had to go all the way up Sabino Canyon Road and come in through some horse trail or something. ..."

"Yup, that's the one."

"God, it was a dump back then," I said.

"It's worse now," he said. "But the price might be right."

Enid and I made a date to go take a look.

We drove up the driveway to the ranch and couldn't help but notice that everything was dilapidated and in disrepair. We parked in front of the ranch house and were greeted by the owner, his son and his daughter-in-law. It really was a dump.

After a quick look inside the buildings, we went out to walk the property. We had barely taken 20 steps when we looked at each other and smiled. A covey of quail ran out in front of us, crossing our path. It was spring, the birds were chirping, and the view of the Santa Catalina Mountains was spectacular. Enid and I could feel the energy of the land.

Ever stand some place and know that the ground is special? Sacred somehow? That's what happened to us that day. As we walked back on the flagstone path toward the old pool, we started to talk at the same time, using the very same words: "Do you feel the magic?" It was odd, because at that point in our lives, neither of us was the spiritual type. But magic was what we felt. Energy. And amazingly, this magic plot of land was right in our backyard—I hadn't realized it before, but the Double U actually backed up to our property on two sides. It was our first and last stop in our search for a place to build our fantasy resort. Three weeks later the 42-acre Double U Dude Ranch was ours, 16 horses and all. (Those I gave away.) The asking price was $750,000, the owners kept a few items, and we settled at $714,000. It took us until September to get all the principals together, and we closed escrow the day after Labor Day. We decided to call our place Canyon Ranch.

CHAPTER 8

Creating an Oasis in the Desert

From day one, I envisioned Canyon Ranch as an "oasis in the desert," embracing and lush, with water running through it. The rest of the world saw dirt and cactus and rocks. But I saw green, a patch of rest and rejuvenation in the middle of miles of dry, hard landscape. I remember saying, "We're going to get Midwesterners and East Coasters—we can't have a stark, barren stretch of desert."

If you look around the property today, you'll see exactly what I imagined as I stood in the middle of the old Double U. So help me God, I could visualize everything in precise detail. I knew just where I wanted to put the new buildings and the lawns, where the new trees and bushes would go, and how I wanted the buildings to be framed in greenery. I knew where I'd put a fountain, a stream, a pond. I wanted to hear the tranquil sound of water flowing through the grounds. And of course, since I owned the local water company then, it was easier for me to think about how to pay the water bills.

By the time we actually completed the purchase, I was well under way with architectural drawings and layouts for new buildings, an expanded ranch house (later we'd call it "the clubhouse") with a new entrance, and a novel design for a 28,000-square-foot spa and exercise building. It would be huge—unlike any gym or sports facility yet built. I'd spent the summer thinking and sketching, usually watching a baseball game at the same time. I was good at floor plans, understanding how people used and moved through space.

Enid and I had a vision of how the spa and public spaces should look and feel inside. The tones and furnishings would be soothing, soft greens, beiges, neutrals—a warm desert palette. There'd be artwork on the walls of the gym, and natural wood and tile on the floors. We'd manage the sound too. You'd hear the twitter of our birds and the burbling of the creeks, not the pounding of exercise machines or nearby traffic. Our resort would be a space for healing. Nothing bright, noisy or shiny to jangle the spirit. No glitz for us! Every detail of Canyon Ranch had to convey that this was a place of restfulness, mindfulness and protection. We'd never seen anything like it, but then, neither had anyone else. We didn't know it at the time but we were inventing modern "spa style." Elegantly simple, earthy, with overtones of Zen.

A gifted architect named John Campisano, who had joined my company five years before, set to work furiously translating my vision. From the first day John and I met, we were design soul mates. He could take my rough sketches and verbal visualizations, put them on drafting paper, and render them overnight in precise architectural detail. Now, I was asking him to do that at warp speed. With his designs, and the help of a draftsman, we got about 150,000 square feet of buildings to the blueprint stage in three months, record time for even a routine development project.

"You lost more than weight at that fat farm!"

Things had gone so well from the moment we'd started planning the resort that I'd hardly thought about financing it. The banks had always been comfortable giving me 80% loans for new real estate ventures, and I had no doubt that I'd find the money for this project just as I had for every real estate project I'd ever developed. So when I made the rounds to talk to bankers this time, I was stunned. Nearly everyone gave me the cold shoulder. This wasn't a normal real estate project, and obviously, they couldn't wrap their minds around what this resort was going to be, and I couldn't adequately explain it. The moment I said I wasn't going to serve alcohol, one of the bankers stood up, all 6'5" of him, and said,

"Zuckerman, you lost more than weight at that fat farm! You lost your f-ing mind."

The only place that would give me a commitment was the one bank that didn't ask me to fully explain the project. It was a local savings and loan that I had done business with for several years, and the bankers didn't care about the specifics—they simply believed in me. "Mel," they said, "if you think it's going to be good and will succeed, that's good enough for us. How much do you need?"

I said I thought I needed $3 million, but I asked for $4 million just to play it safe. I had a couple of million of my own that would get the project going.

"We'd advise you to wait as long as you can before you sign the commitment," they told me, "because interest rates are coming down." Once a commitment is signed, the interest rate is fixed, and a lower interest would save me a bundle of money. So we sealed the deal with a handshake, and I waited for the rates to drop. With the verbal commitment in place, I felt comfortable starting construction with my own money. By my calculation, I would run out of liquid funds just as interest rates dropped, and then I'd start drawing down my loan.

Laying the groundwork

One of the first big decisions we had to make at the old Double U was whether to keep the original buildings. They were square, squat and ugly, and the cheapest, easiest thing to do would be to put a blade to the earth and bulldoze the entire physical plant. But when I thought quietly about leveling the ranch, I worried that I might damage the energy of the property and chase away the wildlife. It wasn't a matter of money. We didn't want to disturb the sacred earth or its inhabitants. I also felt that the old buildings were part of what made the ranch comforting and supporting. Our vision didn't seem to call for brand-new; it should evoke the history and feeling of the Old West. We wanted to create an intimate, restful and rustic setting where guests were encouraged to look inward. A home away from home where they could put their feet up and feel at ease.

But there was precious little in the old shacks that we could salvage, and rebuilding them was an expensive proposition. We jackhammered foundations, ripped out the old wiring and plumbing, and laid new pipes and conduits for electrical wires. None of the existing systems could accommodate our plan. Since we were a mile away from the county sewer, it was an engineering challenge to manage the hookup so that the sewer water flowed downward and in the right direction. We dug trenches that were 30 feet deep and had to reinforce the sides to ensure that there wasn't a cave-in. Our construction estimates rapidly went north.

My son Jay came over from my home-building company to run the renovation of the residential units and build the new ones. We hired a general contractor to handle the two larger buildings. Jay was all of 23, and he loved construction. I was spending most of my time holed up in my office about five miles from the ranch, poring over plans, budgets and timelines, or out on the lot resolving the millions of unexpected problems that come up on a construction site. The summer heat was a killer.

At the same time, we needed to think about what kinds of programs we'd put in all those new buildings. And on that front, I had a running start. Before I'd left the Oaks in April '78, I'd talked to Karma about my plans to open a spa. "Karma, I'm really serious," I told her. "Would you ever consider leaving California and moving to Arizona and coming in with me?"

"In a heartbeat," she said.

She had spent only four weeks working with me, she didn't know me as a businessman, and she had no assurance that I could pull off this venture. Following me into it would be a big risk for a single mom with two young children. But Karma had come to Tucson. Enid invited her to a surprise party for my 50th birthday the month after I returned, and in October she moved down permanently. I've asked her what made her take a chance on me and on my fantasy. She says she somehow knew instantly that Mel Zuckerman and his crazy concept would become "the future of the health and healing world." And the timing was perfect for her. She had been contemplating her next career move, and she didn't see much growth opportunity at the Oaks. Another restless soul! She set to work designing our fitness program.

What f-ing magic did I feel on the ranch in the crazed middle of August? Magic or one heat-stoked mirage? At that point, I could have gone either way. I was supercharged with the idea of my new project, but what if I was wrong? Over the course of the summer, before the sale closed, I got into a pissing contest with the Double U owners. It was over an old car worth less than $5,000. The car was part of the corporate assets, which we had bought in full, and I thought we could use it to run some of our errands during the construction phase. The old owners didn't want to give it up. "They're being difficult," I complained to Enid, who was away in San Diego. "This car could blow the whole deal."

"Forget about the car," she said. "Stop looking for a way out."

She was right. I did have cold feet. And hearing the truth from her got me back on track. (Again.)

Welcome to the insanity

I'd turned the financial end of my home building business over to a guy named Jerry Cohen, who'd long been one of my favorite bankers. We had an easy camaraderie, and earlier in the spring, still fresh from Ojai, I had dropped in to see him. I wanted to tell him about two new business ideas: starting a new professional basketball team in Tucson and building a fat farm, "like the one where I lost all this weight." He rolled his eyes a little. The next time I saw him, he said, "I like one of your ideas ..."

"You like the basketball team," I said.

"No, actually, I like the fat farm," he said. "That one has a chance."

Jerry and I both loved sports. But unlike me, Jerry believed that a professional sports team couldn't be successful in Tucson because the University of Arizona dominated the local sports scene, especially in basketball. He turned out to be right. The basketball team I started at the same time folded, as did the new league, after one year. But my Tucson Gunners won the league championship, and it was fun—expensive fun.

Just about the time we broke ground on the ranch, Jerry's bank was sold, and he was out of a job. Jerry was a CPA, just as I had been in my earlier life, and we were a good match. Two accountants with the same approach to numbers. I brought him into my building operation, and he has been my right hand ever since. Jerry was instrumental in winding down my home-building operation, and he has been a major player in every significant management and operating decision at Canyon Ranch ever since. Literally, I couldn't have gotten Canyon Ranch up and running without him at my side. Later, as we became successful, he became my partner in all Canyon Ranch ventures. But that long, close history may seem surprising given what I threw him into at the beginning. You could say it was trial by fire.

We had given ourselves an opening date of October '79, so we were fast-tracking and burning through my personal funds. By March, four months into the project, I was close to the point where I needed to use the loan I'd lined up to pay my construction crews and keep them working. Thankfully, as predicted, interest rates had come down slightly. But just when we really needed the money, I got a phone call from my friendly banker. It was the worst of bad luck. My S & L was owned by a holding company that also owned a commercial bank, and new federal regulations required that it get rid of one or the other. The holding company had chosen to jettison the S & L, and immediately set a limit of $250,000 on new mortgages.

My buddy at the bank was almost in tears. "Mel, I don't know how to tell you this," he said, his voice quivering. "We can't make the loan."

I stopped breathing for a moment. Part of that $4-million loan was supposed to cover our start-up and working capital. We were running on empty. But even then I had a sense of humor. "Bob, quick! How about making me 16 little loans instead?" I knew it was a joke. I was basically screwed.

Bob the banker said he'd do anything he could to help. Some New York banks were considering moving into Tucson, and he would try to get a consortium of them together to participate in the loan. But the idea didn't go anywhere. Interest rates had started moving sky high again, and they were going up all the time. The banking community was in a panic, and all the banks ceased expansion plans. The prime rate ultimately hit 21%. My brilliant strategy of waiting to sign those loan papers turned out to be the biggest mistake of my business life. In 1992, Harvard Business School did a case study on Canyon Ranch that concluded, "Zuckerman acted totally irrationally, starting without a signed commitment." Rationality has never been my strong suit, but fortunately I've always been pretty good at getting back on my feet.

My back to the wall

I was in too deep to consider stopping. But I was out of cash. Jerry was close to hysterical. "We're done. Close it down. Stop everything!" I thought about what he said. In many ways, he was the rational voice. It was a financial disaster. Way over budget, the clock ticking, and no funds to speed the work. "I can't stop," I told him. "If we stop now, in a year these half-completed buildings will be covered with tumbleweeds." I decided that whatever it took, I would keep construction going. I'd liquidate everything. I sold my other real estate, though rising interest rates made that difficult, and a lot less lucrative than I'd hoped. I cashed in my investments, drew down all my cash in the bank. The cushion I'd thought would keep Enid and me going financially while we enjoyed our little mom-and-pop health venture? Gone! Totally gone! We had stepped off the financial cliff. The one thing I didn't hock was my water company, and I joked that at least we'd have something to keep us liquid.

A sane man might have admitted defeat and abandoned the project. But I had a wife who held true to the same vision that obsessed me. "Whatever it takes," Enid said. "I believe in you. You'll get it done. You always have. If you have to put our backs to the wall, do it." So I did. From that instant, cash flow was a crisis. We'd get a small loan here or there, use it to pay off some of our expenses, and take out another loan to pay off the first. Thank God for my good reputation!

Of all the bankers in Tucson, only one came to my aid. Jim Click. He was a fledgling car dealer, and with a group he had just bought the bank where Jerry had been working. He came out to our construction site, looked around and said, "How can I help?" He went back to his board and called us to offer us a loan of $500,000. "We believe in you," he said. In those days it was a lot of money, much appreciated at a very delicate moment.

Friends came to me and said, "I hear you're hurting and that your banking commitment fell through. I want to know what I can do to help you through this." Good loyal friends, who went to their banks and borrowed money against their own credit to help me.

Like many hard-pressed operations, we constantly borrowed from Peter to pay Paul. On Mondays, we didn't quite know where we'd get the money for the Friday paydays. Jerry was juggling funds all the time, and we were struggling to keep everyone paid in full so that the project could keep moving ahead. In the end, we paid every single bill to every single person who ever worked for us. But it took awhile.

Time sped forward and we tried to keep up. Construction delays made our October date look like a fantasy. Four weeks before opening, we still had mounds of dirt and pipes to lay. Now, our target was Christmas. That wasn't just a random date. Winter was the high season in Tucson, and we needed to be open for business so we could get some cash flowing back in.

Everyone was feverish from the desert heat and the time pressure. Enid raced to get the décor done for all the public spaces, the spa building, clubhouse and all the guest rooms. Her job was to work with the decorator to design color schemes and select all the furnishings and fixtures. The short lead-time for delivery meant that all her choices had to be final long before the first guest arrived. With Karma, we were interviewing and hiring staff, defining the fitness programs and lending a hand wherever it was needed.

John Campisano huddled over his blueprints, endlessly making adjustments as the plans crunched up against inevitable construction reality. Jay was everywhere, supervising the workers. He and his wife, Jill, had moved into the area of the ranch next to the horse corrals, where they'd combined two or three of the tack rooms into a makeshift apartment. They lived there for a year, and conceived our granddaughter there too. Talk about being productive!

We had no air conditioning, and with the relentless desert sun and saturating monsoons, it was like working in the middle of the Sahara. Jerry was worrying about the numbers and the bills, and I was stressing over every construction detail and planning where every plant and tree should go. So much for my plan to get out of the rat race! It was all hands on deck. No one slept much, and we all pitched in to do whatever was required to meet our deadline.

The crazy thing is, we didn't even know what we didn't know. None of us had ever operated a hotel, and here we were opening a hotel. We were opening a restaurant too, and none of us had ever done that either. We were inventing a new form of resort from scratch. In retrospect, we were hopelessly naïve. We had more guts than brains.

But against all odds, Canyon Ranch opened on Dec. 20, 1979. We had a staff of 88—and eight guests. Number of guests paying full price: One.

Clearly, we were off to a rip-roaring success. There was no money for advertising or PR, and I guess with our ebullient optimism we simply assumed that "If we build it, they will come." But, at least early on, we were wrong.

CHAPTER 9

Mel Zuckerman, President and Bell Captain

———◦•◦•————

M y first Canyon Ranch business card read "Mel Zuckerman, President and Bell Captain." I carried bags, hosed down the driveway, swept the portico. Enid made beds. Karma tried to supervise the kitchen until the chef threw her out and told her never to come back. We did whatever we needed to do to keep the doors open, and we believed that we were going to pull it off. But not one of us had a clue what was in store for us.

In 1980, our first real year in operation, the place was three-quarters empty most of the time. Our average paid occupancy rate—hotel talk for the number of beds we filled— was a whopping 22%. Enid remembers walking into the dining room one evening when there were only four guests. "It would be cheaper for me to take you all out for dinner than to have the dining room open," she joked. Many of the people who came first had been regulars at the old dude ranch and wanted to see what we'd done with it. There was also a high curiosity factor among the crowd that regularly came to Tucson from Chicago to escape the snow. We were the new place in town, a novelty. But the going was slow. On our first Thanksgiving at the ranch, I refused to get out of bed until Enid came in and dragged me out. "We have guests here," she said. "They're expecting you."

It seemed as if the whole world was crashing around us again. Every week, just coming up with the money for payroll was a struggle, a financial juggling act that mostly fell on Jerry. He moved money around so fast to pay our operating bills that I could barely keep up with his dance steps. Nothing was ever illegal, just lightning fast turnarounds with funds from this account to cover that account. Getting Canyon Ranch through each week solvent was an exercise that left him exhausted.

I was exhausted too. But that might have been because I was always jogging and taking aerobics classes on the ranch. By month four, Enid and I had moved out of our house and into two guest rooms on the property—we wanted to be there full time. Partly that was so we could work, filling in for the hotel manager, making beds, clearing tables, noticing trash that hadn't been picked up or talking to a guest who was in need of support. But at the heart of it, we had gone through all this grief because we wanted to fully participate in the Canyon Ranch lifestyle—eat the food, use the gym, go to the classes, get the massages—and so we did. Long before we ever sold our "real" house and built a new one on the property, we were living full time within the Canyon Ranch bubble, committing our lives to the principles our new fitness resort would preach.

Our earliest guests, though they weren't numerous, were happy, even wildly enthusiastic, and they told their friends. Word of mouth spread. That was good news since word of mouth was our sole marketing strategy, and the only one we could afford. Getting raves from our visitors wasn't hard because our staff was first rate. Karma had had near perfect pitch in putting together the fitness team. She, Enid and I had vetted each candidate, and the three of us had had the tough duty of road testing their skills, which meant daily massages from those competing for spots on the new Canyon Ranch massage team. We'd lived in Tucson for 20 years, but until we placed an ad for body workers in the paper, we hadn't realized there was a whole community of people—healing arts, alternative culture types—who had settled around Tucson because they, like us, were drawn to what they felt in the land. There were a lot of talented teachers and healers— in a lot of tie-dyed clothing—out there.

Jerry, Enid and I teamed up to assemble the rest of the staff for managing the hotel, running the dining function and keeping up with landscaping, maintenance, housekeeping, cleaning, as well as all the other day-to-day headaches of running a 42-acre, 66-room campus as a fitness resort. For comparison, today we have 190 rooms plus approximately a hundred houses and condos covering approximately 175 acres. And a total staff in Tucson of 750 to 900 depending on the season.

To begin with, our program was pretty conservative: gyms with cardio equipment (mostly treadmills), a weight room, five studios for group exercise classes, pools, tennis and racquetball courts, a walking trail, massage rooms, Jacuzzis and a steam room. Nothing very much on the fringe. High exercise, low calorie consumption and clean desert air. But even in our earliest days, we were drawn to innovation.

Boot camp for fitness instructors

Karma embodied the approach to fitness that had changed me, and I turned her loose to create a program in her own image. As she pulled together her team, it wasn't enough for her that the fitness instructors be certified as trainers. They had to demonstrate a gift for the work, and be willing to let her train them, even if it meant going against previous professional training they had received. Working at an off-site gym, she molded her team according to her own instincts of what fitness should be, not what had been taught in physical education programs. She sent her recruits out into the shopping malls of Tucson for a "Seeing the Body" program where they were required to watch how people moved their legs or hips, how they used their hands and feet. She wasn't interested simply in training people to teach aerobics; she wanted them to understand the human body and how it moves.

She was as hard on her new team as she'd been on me. She worked her people in grueling sessions, running through the Tucson heat, in class until 9 or 10 at night. Some recall that time as boot camp. Each staff member came away physically fit enough to lead the menu of class options she'd devised, and understanding the "right way" (Karma's way) to teach them. Karma invented what is now the Canyon Ranch fitness style: how to open and to close each class, how to dress right—it was Lycra leotards, lipstick and neatly combed hair for the women, gym shorts, T-shirts and a tight shave for the men. The uniforms left no place to hide spare body fat or lagging muscles, so there was a powerful incentive for the instructors to be in top form.

Most important, Karma created the template for how to educate and interact with the guests. It was all about finding ways to reach people like me. The ones with a lot of desire, but no faith they could change until someone took the time to show them how. This was the beginning of treating fitness instruction as a profession, and our fitness staff established a level of excellence that continues to make us proud.

But Karma's vision, and ours, was larger than that: Even the most straightforward-looking exercise classes were designed to help people discover the power of possibility.

The scientific method

From the beginning, Enid and I wanted the bedrock of the ranch's programs to be science-based, not "la-la, woo-woo." We wanted to make sure that what we offered was always informed by the cutting edge of research and geared to the education of the guests. We recruited two important mentors from the University of Arizona to assist us in developing the education, nutrition and behavioral change components for Canyon Ranch: Dr. Jack Wilmore, an exercise physiologist, and Dr. Gail Harrison from the Department of Nutrition. Jack's job was to work with Karma and analyze each one of our fitness classes to be sure that all the movements were safe and effective for joints and muscles. Gail looked at all the original menus and recipes that our first menu planner, Jeanne Jones, had developed, and her staff assessed each dish for the calories and nutrition each serving delivered. Together, Jeanne, Gail and our chef created the idea of a healthy menu with enough choice and flavor to be tantalizing, but still within tight caloric restrictions.

Take a hike

As aggressive as we were about finding people to help us flesh out our original vision, I think our real skill was in accepting good ideas and good people when they fell into our laps. Looking back, I think I was a good listener—and I wasn't afraid to act on what I heard.

When we were still in the throes of construction, a peppery New Yorker who had recently moved to Tucson bustled in to see me. Her name was Phyllis Hochman. As part of her own recovery from a back injury, Phyllis had fallen in love with hiking and with the mountains and canyons surrounding Tucson. She'd joined a local hiking club full of hikers of all ages, from 20-year-olds to 80-year-olds, and taught herself everything about the terrain, the desert cacti and shrubs and the desert wildlife. She'd heard that we were building some kind of spa resort and she wanted in.

"I want to be your trail guide," she said.

I looked at her. "What's a trail guide?"

"I lead hikes," she said.

"We're a fitness resort and we're going to have fitness classes," I told her. "We don't have a hiking program."

Not missing a beat, she shot back: "You do now!"

She handed me a proposal that began: "Would you go to Paris and not see the Eiffel Tower?" She was feisty and firm, and I realized almost instantly that she might be right.

After all, we were in the middle of some of the most spectacular desert scenery in the world, and as I was beginning to understand from my own first forays up Sabino Canyon, hiking the trails was both excellent for the body and rejuvenating for the mind. I don't think I would have used the phrase "spiritually uplifting" at that time, but that's the definition of an early morning hike through the Santa Catalina Mountains or Sabino Canyon. There is no better escape from the world than the quiet of such places. And that experience is what Phyllis was offering Canyon Ranch.

There was only one problem: We didn't have a budget for a hiking program. No problem, Phyllis said. She and the hiking guides would work for free. If it turned out to be a popular program, I could re-budget and start paying them. It was an offer I could hardly refuse.

We put a handwritten sign-up sheet on the bulletin board offering four short hikes of two to four miles each. If someone signed up, Phyllis went hiking with them. If no one signed up, she went home. She ran the program for free for many, many months before I could re-budget, using a team of volunteers from her club, who, thank goodness, just loved to introduce people to their passion. Hiking bloomed like a desert flower, and our guests, many of whom came here to deal with emotional issues as well as physical ones, loved their time in the mountains and canyons, communing with the natural beauty. Today, hiking is Canyon Ranch's most popular outdoor activity, staffed by a team of more than 35 outdoorsy full- and part-time guides, and Phyllis, though retired, is still out there walking the trails.

Hiking was the first of many Canyon Ranch activities that seduced the mind into thinking it was on vacation while the body was hard at work, a core principle of the original Canyon Ranch concept. Still, as sure as I was that the program was a good fit for us, I was still amazed to see how it took off. Today hiking is so mainstream that it's become one of the classic family vacations. But 30 years ago, when we first sent people off into the desert with laced-up boots, a knapsack and a light lunch, it was revolutionary. Back then, a lot of people still thought of it as a weird and lonely thing that only backpackers and lost souls did. But in the safety of a resort, we discovered, people were willing to take a chance on something new. We helped make a lot of non-mainstream things very mainstream by introducing them to people who wouldn't have thought of trying them otherwise. We found that with a little encouragement from us, our guests were open not only to body work, but even a foray into the metaphysical. We surprised ourselves by stepping into unexpected realms, and so did they.

Metaphysics, here we come

Astrology came to us when Karma told me about a woman named Nancy Bissell who felt that Canyon Ranch needed her gifts. At first, like any normal CPA, I was skeptical. She did what? Astrology? Please! We're doing serious work here! We were in the fitness business, and I didn't need any help predicting the future: Get some exercise, lose weight and take some healthy habits home and you're on your way to a better life. That's all the fortune-telling people really needed. But Karma begged me to let Nancy do a reading for me.

When Nancy called, she asked if I'd ever had an astrology chart done. "Of course not," I said. "Well, let me come out and show you how it works," she replied.

I couldn't see any downside. Like anyone else, I was curious to see if there was anything she could tell me that went beyond the scam artists on the boardwalk who say you'll go on a long trip or inherit a mysterious fortune. So in mid-February we sat out in back of the clubhouse under the big mesquite tree. She didn't know me from Adam, and she didn't know a lot about Canyon Ranch other than what she'd heard in the community about this crazy guy building a fat farm resort. She asked me for a simple handwriting sample, and the place and time of my birth. She said she'd come back with my chart.

A few weeks later, she brought me a four-page, single-spaced bible of personal insight that I've turned to time and time again over the ups and downs of the last 30 years. Turns out, I'm a Gemini, with fire predominating.

Quoting from her reading:

"Fire symbolizes radiant energy, enthusiasm, inspiration and excitement. Fiery people inspire others with their bold visions. They keep going long after others have dropped; they thrive on risk and adventure. ... Your chart suggests impulsiveness, hastiness, impatience and a tendency to blind action [Aries rising, ruler Mars in Aries]. On the other hand, there is an extraordinary ability to accomplish anything you set out to do. ... Having a dependable network of supportive people to help you is an important check on your impulsiveness. You like to figure things out, you enjoy problem-solving (and probably create large-scale problems to satisfy the need for big challenges in life)—since small-scale activities quickly produce boredom."

It was accurate—disturbingly accurate—and deeply insightful. I couldn't deny a word. I have read and re-read her reading for me dozens, perhaps hundreds of times, over the last three decades. It was a turning point for me, an instant where I became open to a whole set of experiences that I would have dismissed without a serious thought. As fringy as the idea of having a staff astrologer had sounded to me at the outset, if my reading was any indication, it might be a good thing to offer our guests. The Metaphysical Department at Canyon Ranch was born, with Nancy Bissell as our "metaphysician" in chief.

Our metaphysical staff expanded to part-time astrologers,

psychic readers, tarot card readers and intuitives, and they've proven to be talented healers and spiritual guides whose gifts have illuminated complex personal paths for many of our most skeptical guests. Personally, I am still more comfortable with our programs that exercise sinews rather than spirits, but I acknowledge that many, many guests have experienced life-changing moments with our metaphysical department. They have often written to me telling me how they have discovered a spiritual side of themselves here that they'd never before been open to experience. In that realm too, Canyon Ranch was a safe space for exploration and personal growth.

It all comes down to people

Our vision was evolving in ways I never would've expected—and a visit to Canyon Ranch, even in its earliest days, was worlds away from any fat farms or spas we'd ever seen. Guided by our guts and our willingness to take a chance on the inspirations, from whatever source that came our way, we were laying down the central tenets of the Canyon Ranch culture. Enid and I were the "tastemakers," but it was our first 80 staff members and the first few hundred guests who established the core experience. Our governing philosophy was to find the best people we could, train them well and treat them with dignity and respect. We assumed, in turn, that they would treat our guests the same way. It was a good philosophy for hiring and retaining the best talent.

Building on my experience with Karma at Ojai, we aspired to create an environment that was truly loving and nurturing. Love, funny to say, was part of our business model. We hired people who had the ability to make that human connection with another person who might be in need. We understood, and this was especially true early on, that many people who would come on this type of vacation might be very wounded, needy people—just like the Mel who'd wandered into the Oaks—whether they knew it or not. We had to have a staff, professionals and non-professionals both, composed of individuals authentically invested in the culture of helping and healing. Today, the hospitality industry is finding out something we knew intuitively 30 years ago: Genuine hospitality is more than offering a room with a gorgeous view or thick towels at the spa. At heart, it's about love, caring, spirit, compassion and intuition.

As we built our staff we looked for experience and technical knowledge. But we hired people for their humanity. We were never about being a five-star hotel, or a fantastic restaurant, although we have tried hard to achieve a high level of excellence in everything we do. What we prize is our mission: changing lives for the better and giving our guests tools and inspiration to "take home."

One of our maids in the early days was a quiet, busy woman who did her job very well and without a lot of words. For weeks she cleaned the room of a woman who had come to

Canyon Ranch to stop smoking. (That was before we became a non-smoking facility). Every day, there would be fewer cigarette butts left in the ashtray, and finally, there were only two or three. On the day the ashtray was empty, still shining from being cleaned the day before, the guest returned to her room to find a small bouquet of wildflowers and a personal note. A silent gift from a kind woman who noticed.

We didn't always get it right. What looked good on a resume or even in an interview didn't always work out in person. At the start, a lot of people, especially the ones with experience in traditional hotels, didn't understand what we were really about, and how we were different. The guy we hired to be our first general manager was fired before we ever opened. Our opening general manager lasted less than three months. I think we went through eight hotel managers and at least as many spa directors in the first 10 years. But somehow we made it work.

The Love Machine

I used to give talks, short inspirational lectures, to the guests after dinner. One night, six weeks or so after we opened, a man in the audience raised his hand. He was a hotelier with three properties, and he said he had always had trouble getting his staff to his desired level of service and friendliness in less than two or three years. "Your staff is already outstanding on both counts!" he said. "How did you do it? Do you have a special kind of training program?"

For a second, I was speechless. Other than Karma's program for the fitness department, the rest of our training was, to put it generously, minimal. We were nowhere near creating a human resources department. But, the question had been asked, and I had to think fast. The only thing I could do was to make up a funny story, because I was too embarrassed to tell him the truth—it would have made me sound too much like the seat-of-the-pants beginner I was.

"Let me tell you why I think our staff is so good," I told him. "First of all, my wife and I personally interview every key employee; and second, I'm a sort of amateur inventor—I've invented this little finger cuff that detects human emotions. When I have a potential new hire, I slip on the finger cuff. On the wall, I have two lights: One's red, and one's green. During the interview one of the lights goes on. If the red light goes on, I stop the interview right there, and I say thank you but no. If the green light goes on, I hire them."

There were about a dozen people in the audience, and they all looked at me quizzically.

"Yeah?" the hotelier said. "You hire if the green light goes on, and you don't hire if the red light goes on ..."

I smiled. "You know, I call my invention 'The Love Machine.'"

The group lit up. They got it. I explained that the ranch

staff was full of people who were so connected to the mission of improving people's lives that they could give to the guests from an emotional resource that few can consciously tap when they are simply required to perform a task. And then I said, "My little machine detects that capability."

The Love Machine story became a Canyon Ranch legend. On the ranch's 25th anniversary, we had a big thank you party to honor the staff, and at the end of the evening, the staff made a formal presentation to Enid and to me. The lights were dimmed and a group of men came out wearing yellow hazard suits and wheeling a gurney with a small hump on it, also covered in neon-yellow hazmat cloth. Gingerly, the men lifted the cloth, unveiling a little red box with a red light, a green light and the words "Love Machine" painted on two sides. This, our engineering supervisor announced, was "the first Atomic Love Machine."

That "machine," or something like it, has been running constantly since we opened. And as far as I can tell, there's no way we could ever turn it off.

Time and again, when guests write me to glow about their experiences with us, they don't mention the fabulous facilities or the beautiful scenery. They tell me about how one individual staff member—or many—guided or inspired them to a transformation. From the first days of Canyon Ranch we have worked to hire people with natural kindness and with genuine generosity of self, who believe in our mission, buy into it, connect to it and want to make a difference in others' lives. If I could, I would patent the Love Machine and sell it to every service business in America. "Put love first" is really a pretty simple rule to follow.

CHAPTER 10

A Start-Up on a Shoestring

For the first three years, Canyon Ranch was a start-up on a shoestring. When we opened our doors, we still had unpaid construction bills of approximately $1.5 million. The struggle to stay ahead of our bills and keep going and growing was constant. There were times when we almost gave up. People would offer us half of what we had put in to take us out of our misery, but we always knew that we were in it until the bitter end, even though money was short and new financing was impossible to come by. During the first 10 years, I never took a dollar in salary.

My mind often circled back to a conversation I'd had with Sheila Cluff before I left Ojai. I'd told her that I was thinking of opening a place like hers, and she'd been free with her advice. "Let me give you a hint," she said, "You can't spend more than $2 million creating a business like this. Preferably less. But you certainly can't make it work if you spend more than $2 million."

We spent $7 million getting Canyon Ranch open. And as worried as I was that Sheila was right and I'd set myself up for a big-time fall, I somehow never doubted that I would succeed. I was convinced that people needed what we had to offer.

Our word-of-mouth "strategy" began to work, and slowly, steadily, our reputation started to grow. By the end of 1981, our second full year in business, our occupancy had risen to 55%.

Then, out of the blue, we got an unexpected boost. The April 12, 1982, issue of *Time* magazine had a big piece on the ranch by a writer named Jane O'Reilly. The headline read "In Tucson: Balancing the Triangle of Life," and the story—with vivid photos of our desert setting—put Canyon Ranch on the map. I wasn't happy that O'Reilly called me a "super Type A" and a "hard driving relaxer" (though both are probably true). But I was thrilled that she concluded the article by quoting my personal mantra, "I want to feel like this forever." That's what I had said when I called Enid from Ojai, and that's how I justified every struggle to build Canyon Ranch.

Other national publications followed Time's lead and sent writers and photographers. We were in *Glamour*, *Mademoiselle*, *Money* and *Vogue*, among others. Our phone began to ring with people wanting the Canyon Ranch experience.

Marathon Mel – 26 miles in 4.19

Enid and I were the truest of the true believers in the ranch's wellness lifestyle. I was working out every day, jogging outdoors or indoors on the treadmill, bouncing up and down in the aerobics classes, hiking the mountains and canyons. I was finally thin enough to look good in jogging shorts! So, reveling in my own physical prowess, buoyant with my own boyishness at 54, I decided to run my first marathon. I regularly ran three miles a day and occasionally more. Honestly, that should have been enough for me. But two things collided: my own drive to meet new physical challenges, and our corporate drive to bring our lifestyle and health mission to our own backyard.

In 1982, on the heels of the *Time* piece, we decided to sponsor a fitness event for all of Tucson. Because of Canyon Ranch, people from all over the world were coming to Tucson to get fit and healthy. Shouldn't we share that experience with our neighbors? Our goal was to get everyone in town, whether or not they were regular exercisers, to challenge themselves to do something—walk a distance or run a distance—beyond anything they had ever attempted. We'd call it the Canyon Ranch Fun & Fitness Run. It grew into a sort of "How to Run" program, where we encouraged people to set a fitness goal to meet their own personal objectives, whether they planned to run one mile or 26. We'd have a full marathon, a half marathon, a 10K run, a 5K run, or people could choose to walk or jog a mile or two. We even invited mothers pushing baby carriages to come and walk with us. On many Sundays at various local shopping malls, we ran clinics on how to fit running shoes, what to eat before a race, how to train. It was our first attempt to reach out and share Canyon Ranch's mission with our community. The locals still called us the "fat farm" back then.

We had 1,500 participants, and 26 who signed up for the full marathon.

One day in July, I was taking a leisurely jog through Sabino Canyon with my friend Barry, and talking about how crazy people had to be to actually run a marathon.

"Who could run 26 miles?" I said.

"Yeah," said Barry.

"At our age, they would have to be nuts!" I said.

"Yeah," Barry said. "Let's do it!"

It was three months till the marathon, and if we wanted to compete, we'd have to train like madmen. In the heat of summer, no less. At our ages, the recommended training period for a marathon was 18 months to two years. But I was in a phase of my life where I wanted to do things I'd never contemplated doing, and somehow a marathon didn't seem like that much of a stretch. After the first few weeks of training, I started to run 75 miles a week. But my body quickly began to break down. I hurt everywhere. I had to cut back my running to 45 miles a week.

The race day came. I didn't take it very seriously for the first 13 miles. I was full of myself, overjoyed that after never running a single race in my life, I was now in a marathon. In my teeny-tiny running shorts (so teeny I had to tuck my inhaler into my jockstrap), I ran through the streets of Tucson, doing do-si-dos with the crowd. The second half wasn't so much fun. I was in pain, exhausted. But I did finish the race in four hours and 19 minutes, which pleased me no end. My goal had been to run an average of 10-minute miles, which would have been a 4:22. I was right on target, and I might have been able to shave a tad off my time if I hadn't been a fun-squad motivator during the first few miles.

I limped through the days that followed. My doctors think it's possible that by training so hard in such a short time span, I permanently injured my joints. I feel some of those aches and pains to this day. Perhaps I was a fool to run a full marathon in the first place. But I'm so glad I did.

The next year, I was smarter. I signed up for the half marathon of what was to become an annual Canyon Ranch fitness event. Today, it seems that every charity sponsors a run, but in 1982 it was a novel idea to support and empower people like me, with different physical conditions and limitations, encouraging them to do things they had never done before. I'm still proud that at 54 years old, in my first race ever, I ran 26 miles in one stretch! Talk about feeling empowered!

Pressures of growth

It became clearer and clearer to me that in 1982 we were going to be a success. Long before I had the statistics to back up my conviction, I knew it in my gut. But if we were going to make the most of the moment in the spotlight we'd gotten from *Time* and our big Tucson event, we needed to grow. Like the typical entrepreneur I was and am, I believed in the future success of Canyon Ranch long before I could impress anyone else with hard facts.

I estimated that we needed to build at least 10 more rooms, just to accommodate the people we were turning away in the high season. But interest rates were still sky-high, hovering between 16% and 18% for new money, and we were paying 5% over prime on our largest loan. Our interest expense was killing us. With our national profile rising, we were starting to see light at the end of our long tunnel, but we had no idea how we'd reach it. It was a classic small-business problem: We were positioned to grow, but we didn't have the money to do it without giving up ownership in the ranch. And we knew it was too early to even think about that. As usual, we were up against the wall. Somewhere, I had to find someone who could help us.

Savior in the steam room

People often ask me how we've managed to survive all these years. And sometimes I look up at heaven and say,

"Somebody up there likes me." I don't know how or why, but as we went along, people just came out of the woodwork to lend a hand. People like Brown Badgett.

On a trying day in January 1983, Jerry and I had spent hours finessing our finances. It exhausted me, and I figured that the steam room was a sanctuary where I could sweat out some short-term solutions. It was so steamy in there that I couldn't see anything except the vague shape of another body in the room. I went in, spread out my towel and sat down. In gracious innkeeper mode, I naturally said, "Hello." And a voice so raspy that it cut the steam like a serrated steak knife answered me back.

"You look familiar," its owner said.

"It's probably because my face is plastered on a lot of places around here," I said, explaining that I owned the place. My steam room companion started telling me how much he liked the ranch and everything we were doing. He was there with his wife, and she loved it too. He said they were staying for three weeks, although he'd have to fly back home to Kentucky for a few days and would come back again to Tucson to pick up his wife. He had his own jet, though I didn't know it then.

Brown Badgett described himself as "a little ol' poor boy from Kentucky." An old coal miner he was, but he now owned the biggest open pit mine in Kentucky plus a lot of other businesses. He wasn't exactly my type. He was bragging a little, telling me about how he was on the TVA (the Tennessee Valley Authority), how he knew the governor, and how he was a big fan of the basketball team at the University of Kentucky—and knew the coach. I was getting turned off, and I was glad to be able to say I had to go for my massage.

Badgett was waiting for me in the spa lobby when I came out. "I really like you," he said. "How'd you like to see a great basketball game?"

He wanted me to fly to Kentucky with him on a Friday, see the game on a Saturday and come back to Tucson after the weekend. It was to be the biggest game of the year between Kentucky and Houston. Both teams were contenders for the national championship, and he had the best seats in the arena. Badgett was spinning stories of how great it would be. I'd get to see his coal mine and some great horse flesh, maybe even the horse that had won the Kentucky Derby a few years before.

I was completely uninterested. It was cold in Kentucky—like 7 degrees in January. I didn't even own an overcoat anymore. Besides that, I was allergic to horses, and why on earth would I want to see a coal mine? But Badgett kept at it. He even offered to get a girlfriend for me, if that would sweeten the deal. I laughed and said, "I'll let you know. I might like to see the game, but"—and here I concocted a lie—"I've got an appointment with my lawyer that I don't think I can change."

I kept thinking about his offer, though. I'd just made a New Year's resolution that I wanted to get myself out of my rut of doing only things that were in my comfort zone. What could be more out-of-my-rut than to go and spend a weekend with this redneck? So, I went back to him and said, "Why not?" He had his plane pick us up the next week for the three-hour flight to Lexington.

It was the weekend from hell. I enjoyed the basketball game, but that was about it. All I had with me was a light sport jacket and a thin sweater vest, and I was freezing in the Kentucky winter cold. I'd figured I wouldn't be outside much, just jumping from the plane to the car, from the car to the house. Wrong.

Badgett did everything possible to show me a good time—but his idea of a good time and mine were night and day. He took me to his mine, a source of his great pride and terrific wealth, and I had no idea what I was looking at. But it sure was a big hole in the ground. Then, he wanted to show me the prize horses at a stud farm just outside of Lexington. He'd arranged for the Kentucky Derby winner he'd mentioned to be out in the pasture for us to see. The two of us were talking in the back of the car as his chauffeur guided the big Lincoln into the parking area of the farm. We hopped out—me in my jacket and sweater vest—and in a flash, the two of them had locked the keys in the car. It was 7 degrees with a sharp wind, and there was no place to take shelter. The chauffeur checked the ground and garbage cans trying to find a coat hanger—something, anything—to pry open the car door. There was no one around, no one to help, and I was so cold that my teeth were literally chattering. Finally we found a little shed with a potbellied coal stove. I kept thinking about Tucson. Blue skies. Sun. I could feel myself getting sick. Finally, the chauffeur jimmied the car door open, and we got back inside. I never even glanced at the horse.

On Monday morning, we flew back to Tucson. Mid-flight, somewhere over mid-Texas, Badgett leaned toward me. "I like you, Zuckerman, and I like what you do," he said in his growl of a voice. "Is there any way I can get involved?"

I was nice about it, cordial and conversational, but I told him I didn't take partners, and didn't intend to.

He pursued it. "Do you need any help financially? Need a loan? What kind of interest are you paying now? If it's high, I could lend you the money to pay it off. "

I was stunned. He was the most unlikely angel. A tall, gawky, gray-haired guy in wire rims from the hills of Kentucky. But this coal miner's son offered to loan me enough money to pay off our $4-million debt at half the interest rate we were paying at the time, and he sweetened his offer with another million dollars for working capital that he was in no hurry to see me return. "Just pay me when you can," he said.

It all happened in an instant. We had the discussion on the plane on Monday, and by Friday, we had the papers to sign in Tucson. It was the most efficient business transaction of my entire life. I asked the lawyer from Kentucky how they managed to get everything done so fast. He chuckled. "When Badgett wants something done," he said, "we just do it."

It's hard to overstate how important Badgett's loan was to us at that moment. The word was spreading about the ranch, the tide was with us, and with this new infusion of cash, we could imagine finally turning a profit by the following year. Badgett and his family remained part of the ranch family for years. We built him a big house on the property, and he'd come with Heidi, his wife, for extended visits several times each year, bringing his grown son and other family members. His own business interests continued to prosper, with a construction and contracting firm that worked all over the South. We repaid the initial loan within three years, but nothing could truly repay him for the exquisite gift of his timing. We were a fledgling business and we might have survived without him—we always figured out a way—but "might" is an important part of that sentence. I really grew to like and admire Brown Badgett. And I could do a perfect imitation of his raspy voice. It made him laugh.

The world catches up

With the new rooms and funding, we were perfectly positioned when *USA Today* did a cover story on us on Sept. 6, 1984, titled, "Resorts to Keep People Thin Are In." The response was enormous, even though the graph on the cover page showed we were a) very expensive and b) only allowed guests to eat 800 calories a day. By 1985, we were the most famous spa in the country. Women were flocking to Tucson, but men were coming too. By the end of 1985, an average of 30% of our guests were males, and a consistent 75% of our beds were filled every night. We'd been in business for only a few short years, but we were creating the template for the wellness industry, a category we had invented in an industry we'd accidentally kick-started.

We'd barely advertised, and hadn't figured out a true marketing or media relations program, but we were getting lots of good ink. Editors didn't know what to do with us, but they liked us. They didn't have an editorial niche for a fitness or health resort, but they kind of knew what a "spa" was, and they stretched and pulled to fit us into the category. I didn't like it. "Spa" meant all the wrong things to me, but I couldn't complain about the number of guest inquiries we were getting now that journalists had discovered us. I called a "spa" a "Special Personal Adventure." Still do.

Simultaneously, there was a revolutionary expansion in the public consciousness about fitness spreading across the U.S. The idea of lifestyle habits and prevention as pivotal to health was going mainstream. Jane Fonda was everywhere in her leg warmers and leotards. *The New York Times*' columnist Jane Brody was writing weekly on health and behavior, and

USA Today began featuring the "Your Health" section every day. New magazines were sprouting up with titles like *Shape*, *Self* and *Women's Health*. It was becoming normal for people to join health clubs and read labels at the supermarket. The vision Enid had jotted down as we drove home from Ojai was becoming the model for a mental shift on Main Street America.

CHAPTER 11

Evolution and Revolution

———◦•◦•◦———

I knew we had a tiger by the tail. An explosion of consciousness about lifestyle, health and fitness was under way, and it wasn't going away any time soon. And, by accident, we were at the leading edge. Within two or three years of setting out, not only had we become pioneers of a fledgling industry, we had also become its gold standard.

It helped that our timing was perfect. By the time we opened in Tucson, long-term scientific research on health and lifestyle habits was starting to bear fruit. Much of that research had been commissioned right after World War II, and by the 1970s and 1980s, the results of these 25- and 30-year double blind studies were hitting the major newspapers—not just the *New England Journal of Medicine*, but the popular press. You couldn't open a paper without seeing something about the connection between lifestyle habits and the chances that people would develop heart disease and diabetes. "Eat right and exercise to live longer and better" was becoming a public health mantra. And it was a huge wake-up call for many American adults.

One study in particular caught people's attention in the mid-'80s. It was a 10-year study of the health habits of people in their 70s, funded by the MacArthur Foundation. Those who exercised a minimum of three times a week for 30 to 45 minutes in each session were in much better shape and enjoying life at a much higher level than those who did not, the study found. And the differences between exercisers and non-exercisers were most spectacular among the elderly. That study became gospel, and it was reinforced by practically every other major piece of research that came along. Almost as a nation, Americans became aware that exercise could keep them living longer, healthier lives with fewer diseases.

As a result, all sorts of people—people who weren't yet old or ill—started thinking, "Maybe I should join a health club." The Reebok and L.A. Fitness clubs opened, along with many others. Gyms, which had been places where guys went to lift weights or play basketball, reinvented themselves as places where women would feel comfortable working out. Even the phrase "working out" was new. Canyon Ranch became the place to go to practice what the scientists preached.

We offered the only immersion experience in the country where the guest became an active participant in his or her own health.

But I knew that there was more to health than exercise and weight loss. When I got home from Ojai and walked into the house, my daughter Amy started to cry. "There's something so different about you," she said as she threw her arms around me. I knew it wasn't just the weight I'd lost or the beard I'd grown. "I think there is something different," I told her. "I think I'm forever changed."

I've always thought that something happened to me in Ojai that had nothing to do with Karma or the running or the pounds I dropped. Something spiritual happened inside me, and I have spent the last 32 years trying to tap it.

From the beginning, as much as I wanted to move people toward health, I wanted them to experience what I had—that sense of profound change. I didn't want to dedicate my life to helping people simply lose weight. I wanted to give them more. We didn't have a word for it at first, but as time went on we began referring to it as wellness—and wellness had to do with not just the body but the mind and the spirit too.

Chasing that idea put us on a path of embracing change instead of clinging to a static sense of what a "fitness resort" should be. We experimented, followed our impulses and let trial and error move us along.

Taking a look inside

One of the people who interviewed with us early on was a woman named Deborah Morris, who was training to be a yoga instructor. She was fun and outspoken, and I found out she'd been doing some sort of talk therapy with people. She wasn't a credentialed person, but she'd done a lot of studying, and she'd been spending time with spiritual teachers. The spiritual stuff didn't mean anything to me, but I liked her. So we created something we called our "attitudinal healing" program and she worked with people who were grieving or facing other kinds of problems. She was so popular that within a few years we had a staff of therapists with Ph.D.'s helping our guests work through emotional pain or questions about the direction of their lives.

Around the same time I decided to hire someone who could do biofeedback. The minute you see that the mind and body are connected and that what you think affects your physical being, you've got something profound. Budgets were tight, but I knew that we needed it at the ranch.

When guests told us about places that had programs they liked, we looked to see if there was a lesson there for us. I'd heard about a place in California called the Ashram run by a woman named Anne Marie Bennstrom, and in 1982 I decided to go there on a vacation. There were 10 people there at a time, hiking, exercising and living together. I recoiled when I found I couldn't have my own room. There was no food, either, just green juice—it was a modified fast. But it was a good group, and I went to a different place in myself than I usually allowed myself to go.

When I got back, I sat down with Karma and Nancy Bissell and said, "I really feel like we're too focused on the physical here." So we put together a test program, limited to 10 or 12 people, called the Self-Awareness Intensive. It had a small staff, and people would do some soul-searching in addition to the usual program of exercise. It was way ahead of its time for a place like the ranch. When we announced it, I got letters saying, "It sounds like a spiritual program. I get my spiritual sustenance from my religion." But we kept it running for a short time, and the couple of dozen people who went through it got a lot out of it. It was one of many tentative steps toward a larger vision.

It pains me to think about the "mind fitness" program we tried. We outfitted a two-bedroom casita—one of the housing units on the property—with tens of thousands of dollars worth of state-of-the-art biofeedback machines and computers, and designed a program that would teach people to control their brain waves, entering states of heightened creativity or deep relaxation. It was an amazing program, and incredibly effective. But it failed because in a beautiful natural setting like the ranch, no one really wanted to spend four or five hours a day indoors, hooked up to a computer. I guess it's some consolation that couple of dozen more people got the training of a lifetime.

We hired a hypnotherapist, a Frenchman named Jean Pierre Marquez, for another pilot program. The big idea was that he'd work with four or five people, helping them look inside to connect with an inner goodness that would help guide them, so they didn't just have to play life by ear. Today, maybe that would be a meditation program. Then, it felt like inner adventuring. That program evolved as Jean Pierre taught stretch classes that shaded subtly into yoga. His voice was hypnotic, and he'd speak during the class, planting positive seeds—affirmations—in people's minds. We called the class "spiritual fitness," always thinking that the word "fitness" might make it seem safer for people to try things, even as we were stretching the boundaries of what fitness could be.

"You are so young," said Anne Marie from the Ashram, referring to the ranch, when she came to visit us in Tucson. "You don't know what you want to be when you grow up yet." I knew she was right. I remember Deborah saying, "You're going to evolve this place continuously because you're going to create a place people can come to every year with a 'Beginner's Mind'"— a willingness to eliminate preconceptions, an openness to the new. A fresh mental slate. And that's what we've done. From the early days of the ranch, we have had guests who return often. We don't want them to come here and spend their time at Canyon Ranch as if by rote, so we encourage everyone to try something new each time they come, just beyond the edge of their comfort zone. Yoga works for you, what about Tai Chi, or Qi Gong? Happy hiking? This time try a bike trip. Or push your skepticism aside for an hour and visit with an energy healer, or go on a shamanic journey. Or just slow down and try a walking meditation. You never know just what will make the connections that will change you.

Lifestyle as medicine

Nothing was untouched by our sense that we could always do more to bring transformation to the people who came to the Ranch. I intuitively knew in 1984 that to reach our guests at the deepest level, our healing staff needed more than dieticians and physiologists, though those professionals were the bedrock of our program. The "ultimate," I thought, would be if a medical doctor gave consultations and lectures about prevention and the power of lifestyle, exercise and nutrition. But when I mentioned the idea to Jerry, he told me that my "ultimate" would be prohibitively expensive.

I expected that. I used to think of Jerry as my "Jiminy Cricket." We'd get up and go for a morning jog, me brimming with ideas, and before I got them out of my mouth, he'd have given me all the reasons why they wouldn't work. He gave me the best advice, rational sane advice. But fortunately, I was too driven to listen to most of his cautions and objections, and I just kept plowing on ahead.

I told him I wanted a doctor on staff, an extra nurse.

"That's going to cost about $300,000 a year," he said. "And we have no idea if anyone will use it."

"Listen," I told him, "I feel in my heart of hearts that having a doctor will add credibility to what we're saying."

Jerry wasn't having it. But the CPA in me knew how to reach the banker in him. "How many guest nights do we have a year?" I asked him, "40,000? Take that and divide it into what this cost will be."

We divided that number by 365 days and calculated that it would cost just $7 extra dollars per guest night to cover the new salaries.

"I'm willing to bet that people won't decide not to come if it costs another $45 a week," I told him. We wouldn't subsidize the service, we'd just build it into the rate we charged. Even Jerry couldn't argue with that. So we hired our first physician, a cardiologist from Baltimore, in 1985, and our medical program grew from there. Canyon Ranch is a different place because of it. It lets us go beneath the surface. We don't just look at the symptoms, we look at the cause. And today, when people work with our medical staff, some of them find healing that had eluded them everywhere else. It has everything to do with dealing with the whole person in a loving, empowering way.

Many kinds of growth

The five-year period from 1985 to 1989 was our most dynamic building period in Tucson. We went from a 66-room resort to 190 rooms, with condominiums and private homes. Every year during this period we added 10 to 30 new rooms. We began selling condos and casitas, and we doubled and updated our spa and treatment facilities. In addition, we built the Life Enhancement Center, the LEC, in 1988 as a retreat within a resort. We could see that we had two types of people now regularly visiting Canyon Ranch. The majority came for a vacation of choice. But a minority came, as I had gone to Ojai, because they needed to. I understood that those people needed more personal attention from us, and warmth from one another. The LEC concept was to create a supportive program for about 40 guests, housed in a separate building with its own dining facilities, meeting rooms and fitness areas. We'd offer these guests an integrated one-week program to foster group support and education. They could stay for as long as they needed to, and make lifelong commitments to a healthier lifestyle. Thousands, by now, have come through the LEC, and they're the closest to my heart in some ways because they remind me so much of myself.

Along with the LEC, we opened the Health & Healing Center, the home base of our health and medical services. Even though we hadn't wanted to be a medical center, a "Mayo Clinic in the Desert," it was obvious that top quality, medically reliable, yet on-the-cusp health care and medical diagnostics and consultations were something we ought to offer our guests as part of their Canyon Ranch experience. Over time, medical doctors across the country began to consider Canyon Ranch as a place where they could explore a new kind of healing practice, a place where science, emotion and spirit all had a place. We began to attract physicians who were strong believers in combining conventional and alternative medicine. Our doctors have come from Stanford, Johns Hopkins and the Cleveland Clinic, and they're a real elite. We really attract innovators with big hearts.

From the start at the Health & Healing Center, our guests could consult doctors with access to advanced technology who might prescribe meditation, or Reiki or acupuncture as well as, or quite likely instead of, drugs. It was an integrated, mind-body-science approach that came to be known as integrative medicine. As Dr. Andrew Weil said in the early days of our Health & Healing program in Tucson, "The hospital of the future will mirror the Canyon Ranch of today." His prediction has come true. Now, many hospitals work to create warm and healing environments for their patients and add the practices of integrative medicine to the practices of conventional medicine.

Today, people come to the ranch in every kind of condition you can imagine. Some are at the top of their game, and just want to keep it that way. Others are in tough shape both physically and psychologically. Elite athletes come to recover, weekend warriors come to get in shape and never-before exercisers come to learn how to take the first baby step. We have mothers, daughters and grandmothers; single men, fathers with sons and husbands with their wives; groups of men and groups of women; and a large percentage of guests who choose to come alone. Some come for a few days. Others check in for weeks and months, hoping to lose large amounts of weight or recover from their dependence on alcohol, food, tobacco, drugs to cope with toxic doses of stress.

For many of our guests, their visits to Canyon Ranch mark the first time they have actually listened to advice about nutrition, the value of exercise and the need to find balance in life. Like all of us, they have heard, read or been nagged by friends and family about the importance of a healthy lifestyle—and tuned it all out. But somehow, "magically," when they come to Canyon Ranch, they finally take the information to heart.

Perhaps it's because there isn't a one-size-fits-all Canyon Ranch wellness plan. We have as many plans and programs as we have guests. Our job is to recognize, humbly, that each individual is on a journey of his or her own.

A day at Canyon Ranch

Now, as when we began, we give our guests a comfortable, but not luxurious, place to sleep, good healthy food and as many choices—for classes, outdoor adventures, educational lectures, health and behavioral consultations, medical tests and personal services—as they are willing to accept. The typical Canyon Ranch guest (as if any of our guests are typical!) takes about four group exercise classes a day and sits in on one or two lectures during the afternoon or evening.

Of course, each guest ultimately makes his or her own choices, and some take six or eight high-energy classes a day, plus enroll in every other activity we offer. But we try to steer everyone toward balance, which means exertion but not over-exertion. After all, we want guests to leave Canyon Ranch feeling lighter of spirit and more comfortable with their bodies than when they walked in the door.

Just the other day I witnessed one of my favorite kind of Canyon Ranch moments. After a class, a group of guests were still clustered on the floor, each one outdoing the others in demonstrating, or attempting to demonstrate, their prowess in a yoga posture back bend. There were six or eight men and women, from their 30s to their 70s, like kids on a playground showing off their cartwheels and handstands, and collapsing in guffaws to the ground. If that isn't a glorious moment, I don't know what is. Yes, Canyon Ranch is a kind of summer camp for adults, but what can be bad about encouraging adults to have the openness of children for new and life-enhancing experiences?

Today a guest might take a 50-mile bike ride, listen to a

talk on "The Human Need for Attention," try Gyrokinesis, Watsu massage or Yamuna body rolling, or refine her golf game. All these things, but no single thing, have become the experience of Canyon Ranch. We know that it may be a run that changes your life. Or a session with an astrologer. Or a hike into a mountain canyon. Or a crucial diagnosis from a physician who can combine the latest technology with energy work. What we've learned to say to our guests is this: We'll meet you right where you are on your path and not try to force you onto ours.

CHAPTER 12

Why Ruin a Perfect Life?

O wners of other well-known spas thought I was crazy to mess with the tried and true "weight loss and pamper formula" that had defined the spa industry through the 1970s. Until Canyon Ranch came along, people had evaluated a place based on how far the needle dropped on the scale and whether the robes in the rooms were ultra-thick. Only a nut, my spa peers said, would start shuffling programs and expectations the way I had. But I'd been told I was crazy many, many times before in the course of my professional life, and I was undeterred.

Our vision of wellness was powerful, and I wanted to spread it around.

Early in our business, long before we were in the black, I started thinking about a second Canyon Ranch location that would be somewhere on the East Coast. By 1983 we realized

that 60% of our clients were from the Northeast Corridor—
Boston, New York, Philadelphia, Washington, D.C. Guests
kept coming up to me in Tucson saying, "We love coming
here, but we'd really love to have someplace closer to home
that we could visit more often, and get to easily by car or
train." I figured that if I didn't get there first, someone else
would, so I started to think about where we might build. I had
real estate scouts lining up locations to visit, and I planned a
three-week trip East in early 1984.

Shortly before I left, I was talking with Wayne Wickman,
a guest from Houston who'd been a regular almost from
the time we opened. Every time Wayne came, we had
lunch together, and this time I mentioned that I was just
about to pursue plans for a second Canyon Ranch. Wayne
exploded. "You've got the best life in the world," he said. "You
weathered the stressful times. Why would you want to ruin
a perfect life?"

It was a fair question with a simple answer.

"Wayne," I told him, "once an entrepreneur, always
an entrepreneur."

A swing and a miss

I waited till April to fly cross-country—I had no intention
of going East during the winter—and arranged to look at
almost every conceivable site for a resort, from southern
New England to New York, Bucks County in Pennsylvania,

the Poconos, Virginia and as far south as the Carolinas and Georgia. The place that captured my heart was in Charlottesville, Va., a one-hour flight from New York, and about a hundred miles from Washington, D.C.

The Charlottesville site was a jewel, beautiful and graceful, and close enough to Washington to ensure easy access for a big chunk of our East Coast clientele. It had a huge Georgian mansion set on a huge plot of land with a pond and swans, and I envisioned it as my Monticello Canyon Ranch with tall pillars gracing the entrance. I could see the buildings, imagine the guests and feel the hum of the dining room. I threw myself into drawing plans, working with architects and imagining how this East Coast location could expand the Canyon Ranch mission. I worked on it for a year, heart and soul.

Everything seemed predestined for success. The state of Virginia and the local city "fathers" were already calculating the tourism dollars and the jobs we'd create. Universities and the health professionals were gaga over our coming to their region. It was a win-win all around. We were working closely with the University of Virginia College of Medicine, hoping to establish the same kind of relationship we had with the University of Arizona in Tucson. Everyone could see how our resort would benefit the community. There was only one minor hurdle: We had to get the majority vote from the local Albemarle County Board of Supervisors.

It wasn't supposed to be a problem, since we had already gotten a unanimous approval from the county planning department. But the board had three supervisors who represented the urban districts, and three who represented the rural county districts. The city supervisors were enthusiastic, but rural ones were afraid that all the cars and traffic coming to our resort would upset their milking cows. There was a deadlock, and that meant no. We'd actually been undone by a technicality. On this board, the chairman could vote only if the property being considered fell in his district—and ours did. He got to cast the vote that knocked us out.

I was devastated. I packed up and went home, and for a short time I put all the ideas of an East Coast Canyon Ranch behind me. A month or so later, there was a new election in Charlottesville, and two of the supervisors who voted against us were defeated, in part because they had opposed our project, which had broad local support. The mayor called and asked us to reconsider. He could guarantee a positive vote, he said. But I'd walked away from Charlottesville and I was done. I don't hold grudges, but when something is over for me, it's over.

VIP's come flocking

I persuaded myself (for a time) that owning and operating one excellent fitness resort was demanding enough for me.

Or, at least, it should have been. Business was growing, and we regularly had a wait list. Even if they had to get on a plane and spend the better part of a day in transit to do it, people were still coming to Tucson from the East Coast.

We'd been discovered. Canyon Ranch was morphing into a premium destination. Celebrities were pouring in from Hollywood and New York, and the titans of industry, finance and real estate development were here too. The guests got a kick out of being in an aerobics class or on a hike with famous people, and so did the staff, but usually I didn't have a clue who was on property unless they made it a point to come over and say hello. It is exciting to meet, or even get a glimpse of, someone famous. For me, though, every Canyon Ranch guest is a VIP, and deserves as much care—and as much privacy—as someone whose name is a household word.

Of course, some celebrities were happy being celebrities. They were delighted to be recognized by fans and interacted warmly with the other guests. That happened even when an agent or a personal assistant had tipped us off ahead of time that the high-profile person was much in need of rest and would be checking in under an assumed name. We'd make careful arrangements to safeguard those stars' privacy, but they would arrive at the ranch, and within hours they would be exuberantly themselves, comfortable in their fame and more than willing to engage.

What? A problem with my hearing?

It was good to be home. I was back in my fitness routine and hiking the beautiful mountains and canyons. I felt lucky, saved from my own excess of entrepreneurship by the shortsighted supervisors of Albemarle County. I was bouncing around the gym, working out on the treadmills and step machines and dropping into aerobics classes to bop and sweat to the music of the '70s. Daily, I'd be stopped in the locker room, or in the dining room, or on the path to my home by happy guests, and I basked in the glow. This had been the whole point of my journey so far—to provide a space where others could learn to experience life fully. The seductions of Canyon Ranch were maturing, and working like a charm.

But I still itched to expand, even though Enid was dead set against a second location. She was afraid of the stress and didn't think that bigger was always better. "How can we be in two places at once?" she asked me. She had a point. Why, indeed, should I ruin a perfect life? But I needed to quench my thirst for the next challenge. After a short hiatus, I was back on the hunt.

I believed that if we were a two-location resort company, it would validate our whole approach and would not only give Canyon Ranch a boost but also be an energizer for the wellness movement. A second location would let us truly go national, and prove that our success in Tucson wasn't a one-shot flash in the pan.

I was back in my element—thinking big, imagination racing. But I still couldn't move full speed—my body wouldn't let me. For a while, I'd been having some problems with my hearing and balance. And when I finally had it checked, the doctors told me it wasn't just the result of aging or being around construction noise for so many years. I had an acoustic neuroma, a tumor on the acoustic nerve to my left ear. It wasn't cancerous, but if it went untreated, the consequences could be dire: It could paralyze my face, even grow into a large brain tumor. The surgery would be delicate because it was so close to the brain, and in fact, it could've cost me my life. I lived to tell the story, but I lost the hearing in my left ear.

The surgeon cautioned me that my recovery would take six months to a year, and I most likely would have a long period of dizziness and fatigue. But I was back at my desk in record time, hiking the trails and canyons and working out within weeks of the surgery. My surgeon was astounded. He also thought I was reckless to be so active so early. But I think he underestimated what can happen when the patient is at the top end of the fitness scale. I attribute it all to the lifestyle I was living, thanks to Canyon Ranch.

As I was recovering, I wondered if the acoustic neuroma hadn't been a kind of spiritual message for me. Maybe the reason I had developed this problem and lost half my hearing was that I hadn't been listening closely enough. Maybe I didn't need to have a second location after all. Maybe enough was enough. We had recently put down a deposit on another site in the Northeast. I called Jerry from the hospital and told him to get our money back. "Stop everything," I said.

A saner man, less restless man might have sustained the thought. But not me. I was driven to prove the power of the Canyon Ranch model. And soon, way too soon for Enid's comfort and my physician's, we were back looking at sites closer to New York, the demographic heart of the East Coast market—New Yorkers were among our most ardent and frequent guests. I'm guessing that we visited every potential resort site in driving distance from New York City or Boston. We wound up in the Berkshires, in Western Massachusetts.

Winter in New England

The naysayers were out again in force when word got out that I was hoping to open a resort in New England or in the Northeast. Had I spent so many years in Arizona that I'd forgotten about winter? Snow? Ice? Shoveling? In the winter, the only successful resort destinations in the Northeast were in Vermont or New Hampshire, for skiing. The Northeast was fine for vacationing in the summer months, but most intelligent Northeasterners followed the sun, flying south to Florida and the Caribbean, or west to California or Hawaii. But I believed I had an idea that would keep them close to home.

My plan was to build an enclosed, four-season resort where guests could come and enjoy the scenery and surroundings, and participate in vigorous healthy activity—regardless of the weather. We'd connect all the buildings, with airy, bright enclosed passageways between guest rooms and dining rooms, pool and gyms, lobby, meeting spaces and treatment rooms. All the public and private spaces would be accessible and inviting, and guests would never have to worry about dressing for the nasty weather. The right site would have the footprint to make that possible.

We found it at the location of the Bellefontaine Mansion in Lenox, Massachusetts. Enid, who had been in New York City, had driven up to see it and called me in Tucson. "I think you should see this place," she said excitedly. Once it had been an elegant, turn-of-the-century mansion. Now it was in close to total disrepair, with a caved-in roof and crumbling internal walls. Only the library had survived the building's travails intact. But the mansion was located on 120 acres of rolling green lawns bordered by a piney forest. Even better, it was right in the middle of the best scenery in the Berkshires. And it was just down the road from the historic town of Lenox, close to Old Stockbridge and near all sorts of cultural sites and activities—Jacob's Pillow, Shakespeare & Company, the Norman Rockwell Museum—and Tanglewood, the summer home of the Boston Symphony Orchestra. For many New Yorkers, the drive to Tanglewood for concerts was a ritual;

a Sunday afternoon picnic on the "lawn" was an annual summer pilgrimage for many. The area was breathtaking.

The Bellefontaine itself was steeped in history. Built in 1897, the grand estate had been a summer residence of the Geraud Foster family until 1945. Then, for a while, it was a monastery. Over the years, it had been rebuilt twice after damaging fires. In 1980, it passed into the hands of a real estate developer from Boston who hoped to transform it into a resort. He'd spent seven years planning the project and getting the town of Lenox's approval to build it—then he'd abandoned it.

Was there a message in that for me? Possibly, but I'd taken one dilapidated property in a gorgeous natural setting and turned it into a winner. Why wouldn't I be able to do it again? As I had at the old Double U Dude Ranch, I could see the finished product from the start, long before contracts were signed or money was lined up. And once again, the process of translating that vision would involve unanticipated obstacles, cost overruns, construction delays and rolled back opening dates. It was Canyon Ranch revisited in more ways than one.

CHAPTER 13

All Hands on Deck

———◆•◆•◆———

Once I had the keys, I discovered that Bellefontaine was even more of a wreck than I'd thought. The old, gracious library and the entrance were beautiful in a turn-of the-century way, but the construction was turn of the 19th century and we needed it to operate for the 20th and 21st century. All the modern updates were terrible, and costly to fix. I wondered aloud, and sometimes to Enid's annoyance, whether we'd be better pulling the whole thing down and starting fresh. I fantasized about setting eight sticks of dynamite under the main building.

We had on-site contractors who managed the construction, but Enid and I zigzagged from Tucson to the Berkshires for inspections, managing one booming but demanding resort while in the throes of inventing another.

What were we thinking when we added this headache to our lives? The stress was constant again.

Construction started in February 1988, and Enid moved to Lenox in July '89, planning to stay right through the opening, which was originally set for late summer. Ultimately, she wouldn't be home until winter. Our summer date moved to October as we delayed and rescheduled our opening six times over eight weeks. I went back and forth from Tucson, but Enid held down the fort, working with the new team members we had hired in Massachusetts, helping them understand what Canyon Ranch standards meant.

We were a tiny core of transplants from Tucson, building a new "family" in the middle of a quiet New England town. We worked side by side, slept in local motels and ate dinner together every night. This time, we weren't flying blind, as we'd been in Tucson. We were old hands who knew our way around the hotel, restaurant and fitness businesses, and we had the reviews to prove it. We weren't cocky, but we figured that since we'd pulled it off once, the second time should be a cakewalk. Our operating assumption was that good people would come out of the woodwork again, just as they had in Tucson.

Of course, Enid and I couldn't interview all the applicants the way we had before—the pressures of operating a spa on the other side of the country meant we had to delegate some of that to our trusted team. And this time around we were opening a facility that had twice the number of rooms as the original Canyon Ranch, and instead of 80 staffers, we needed 250 to open Lenox. And one other thing: Enid and I were both 10 years older. We didn't look or feel it, thanks to our outrageously healthy lifestyle, but it wasn't easy to fend off the stress of starting another venture from scratch and trying to be in two places at once.

The run-up to the opening didn't go as smoothly as we'd hoped. The communities surrounding Lenox just didn't have the same kind of talent pool we'd found in Tucson. The only well-trained department was fitness. Rebecca Gorrell, who had been in the fitness and movement departments at the Tucson resort for several years and had worked under Karma's direction, asked if she could have the role as fitness director in Lenox. She was another great taskmaster. But service personnel had us stumped. At first, we couldn't find people with the appropriate hospitality experience. Tucson, if not a big city, is at least a city. The Berkshires are a collection of tiny New England villages. And the applicants who lined up for jobs weren't prepared to take on the demands of urban guests from New Jersey and New York, or meet the expectations of people who'd already had that touch of Canyon Ranch magic (and dare I say, the "Love Machine"?) in Tucson.

But we did our best to bring the Canyon Ranch culture east. In the days when we didn't yet have a dining staff or a functioning kitchen, every night a group from our Tucson opening team would go to one of the few restaurants that could accommodate our large party. It was fun. Hard work, but a great way of creating the camaraderie that would prove to be so crucial to bringing the Canyon Ranch "culture" east.

Since I'd left the headaches of construction to someone else, staff training was the job of our Tucson team, with me supplying the vision. It was challenging, and by necessity it extended long past the time we opened. We were nowhere close to ready for our first guests, and I knew it. We had planned on a soft opening in August or September with perhaps 20% occupancy and rooms offered at a significant discount so that our staff could learn their jobs without pressure. But construction delays meant the rooms weren't ready that early, and as soon as they were, we had no choice but to have a hard opening, at close to full capacity. If we wanted to get any revenue flowing in before the winter set in, we had to swallow hard and fling open the doors.

People still remind me of the pep talk I gave to help us brace for the looming fiasco. I gathered the entire staff, 250 people, on the indoor tennis court, where most sat on the floor and others stood against the side walls.

"This opening is going to be a disaster," I said, "but it won't be your fault—it's mine. We haven't appropriately trained you, and you are going to be dealing with some of the most difficult guests in the world." I told them that when guests were unhappy, no one on the staff was to take on that negative energy. Guests should be told to "direct all complaints to Mr. Zuckerman."

But mostly, I spoke about the mission and the guests. How they would need love and compassion from the staff, and would need the staff's support. I explained that Canyon Ranch was much more than a resort or a hotel; it was a place for healing. And all staff members, regardless of their specific job, were a crucial element in creating an environment that would help people heal or make the transition to a new life. They would be making a difference in the lives of others, I told them, and they could gain fulfillment from that. It was a good speech. When I finished, there was silence, and I could see tears on the faces of some members of the staff.

Ready or not, here we come

On October 1, 1989, we opened Canyon Ranch in Lenox with 120 rooms, 250 staff members and 75% of our rooms filled. It was a far cry from our opening day in Tucson, with its 88 well-trained staffers serving eight guests.

This birth was a rough one. Our reputation had preceded us, and people had high expectations that we just couldn't meet. There was food and there were towels, but guests often sat down in the dining room only to wait for 15 minutes before anyone offered them a menu. The servers blamed the kitchen; the kitchen blamed the servers. It was chaos, and

New Yorkers have short fuses and low tolerance for chaos on an expensive vacation. I can play back all too many scenes of irate guests dousing the desk managers with invective over how we'd failed. In a way, we'd done it to ourselves. We had this big reputation, and we had placed ads in the *New York Times* that said, "A New Grand Canyon is coming to the Berkshires!"

To our chagrin we discovered that on Sundays, many of the housekeepers assumed that they didn't need to come in. So Enid was making beds again and cleaning toilets, this time for a much larger hotel. She remembers that early on the opening Sunday morning, she treated each guest room as if it were her own—folding the nightgowns, changing all the sheets, plumping the pillows, exchanging all the towels. By afternoon, she was barely patting the pillows into place before rushing on. When one couple, mistaking her for the full-time housekeeper, came into their room and began to complain loudly about "Mr. Zuckerman," Enid said, "Well, I'm his wife!" The guests were so shocked that she'd been pressed into that kind of service that they offered to help her finish cleaning their room—and any others on her list.

It was the worst stress possible. For the first few weeks, whenever anyone wrote and complained about the service, I simply sent them a refund with a note asking them to give us a chance and a few months to get our act together. It was humbling, not being able to deliver our usual perfection, especially since we were right in the backyard of the most habitually critical of all American consumers. Thank God for our "regulars," the guests who came to Lenox after having been to Tucson. They would walk around the spa and the locker rooms and buck up the other guests. "Don't worry about this. You don't know this guy, Zuckerman. He'll make it right. In fact, it will be unbelievable in six months." I gave back the money but these guys were equally generous in disbursing moral support.

We did make it right, but the first couple of months were a nightmare. Enid remembers one winter night when the two of us were sitting in the elegant but almost empty dining room at the Bellefontaine saying, "We are here. We will make it. And we will be the best we can be." We felt as if we were back where we had been 10 years before, in the early days of Tucson. But neither of us ever considered giving up.

Is it getting hot in here?

We were reasonably calm at first, in part because we weren't in a deep financial hole when we opened Lenox. This time I wasn't going it alone. I didn't need to. The Tucson resort had a proven track record, and even better, we had solid financials, and money in the bank. Scores of regional and national banks had begun to approach us to see if there was a way to participate in our success. It was pretty amusing to Jerry and me. We found it ironic that bankers were so willing to offer us money when we needed it the least. They love to make risk-free loans. There were also many well-heeled individuals who had first experienced Canyon Ranch as guests, then become believers in the mission and in us. They had sought me out in Tucson and offered to become our partners or investors in whatever venture we planned next. To a one, they were like Brown Badgett, the Kentucky miner who'd thrown us a lifeline early on: willing to invest big chunks of money with us and get minimal returns on their investment.

But I didn't want partners. I'd never been good at sharing the steering wheel, except with Jerry, who had become my working partner and taken a small share of the business in 1986. I worked alone. I was a vision guy, and the idea of some other potential partner questioning my vision made me very edgy.

So, in addition to the normal first mortgage bank financing of 60% for Lenox, we'd decided to bring in a few limited partners, who'd put in $15 million. They would get a reasonable return on their investments (and some perks at the new resort), but would have no input into operations or management. Still, despite my best-laid plans, and my vow that I'd never again put my own finances at risk the way I had in Tucson, I ended up putting $7 million of my own into the project, almost twice as much as I'd put into getting the original Canyon Ranch up and operating. Our agreement with the limited partners specified that we'd cover any cost overruns, and we were 10% off on our estimates of construction costs. That wasn't a huge discrepancy but it was significantly more than we'd planned. We had also promised the limited partners that Canyon Ranch would cover all operating losses up to $3 million. We weren't really worried, though. Based on our Tucson experience, and our East Coast following, we thought we'd probably break even as early as the first year.

But instead we plowed through our $3-million reserve in the first 18 months, and the losses kept mounting. Even though Lenox had a paid occupancy of 56% the first year, and more than 63% the second, an enviable statistic in the hospitality industry, we were still in the red. Labor costs were 25% higher than we expected, and the toll of winter weather meant that our basic maintenance and utility bills were more than we had imagined. And unlike Tucson, where we had nine months of high season rates and a scant three months of low season rates, in Lenox we had the reverse: a scant three months of high season rates and nine months of low-season rates. Add to that the natural predilection of New Yorkers to demand a bargain, and even with our all-weather physical plant, the New England climate was against us.

For all my confidence that we'd be able to share the financial burden with our partners, we were as much at risk with Lenox as we had been with Tucson. What had happened to the simple vision I'd had for my life on the drive back from Ojai? I puzzled over that for the long, long seasons it took for Lenox to gain momentum.

CHAPTER 14

The Gold Standard

———◆◆◆———

Things actually improved fairly rapidly in Lenox, at least for the guests. The systems started to smooth out and our visitors were happier, some even coming back for the second or third time. Once the operation began to run like a reasonably well-oiled machine, we observed that the Lenox guests often had different needs than the ones in Tucson. They were coming for shorter stays, and with different hopes for what they would accomplish while they were there. They also arrived in a much different state of mind.

Tucson is a destination—most of our guests get on a plane to reach us. That plane trip may be long for some, but it's a kind of decompression chamber that helps ready them for their Canyon Ranch stay. In Lenox, most of our guests just pack up the car and drive to us after a full day's work, or at first light in the morning. No time to make any sort of transition from one mental and energy state to the other, and not as many days to achieve the deceleration. When guests arrive by car in Lenox, you can almost hear their 72-hour clock start ticking down.

Early on, we had the idea that we'd invite arriving guests to spend 20 minutes in a "decompression room," a living room set up with big leather chairs and footrests, and headsets playing relaxing New Age music. The room stood empty. We created "stress tapes" with names like "Letting Go." No one listened to them. But we were onto the nub of a big idea: how to distill the complexities of Canyon Ranch into a transformative, restorative experience for guests with perhaps three days to spend, instead of the average weeklong immersion experience in Tucson.

It was a crucial step in expanding our mission. Over time, I think we perfected our short-form Lenox programs and ultimately allowed Lenox and Tucson to have separate, and equally winning, personalities. It's no accident, for example, that so many of our East Coast guests have come to depend on Lenox as their destination for medical checkups. They needed both the efficiency of having top-flight medical consultations in one site, and the special Canyon Ranch focus that comes from physicians who have the time, training and professional disposition to focus on whole-person wellness. In many ways, our medical program, though begun in Tucson, came to its full fruition because of Lenox.

The more we customized Lenox for our East Coast crowd, the more I could look around the spa lobby and see people smiling and good-humored. Visiting Lenox was becoming a pleasure for me. And though it has never been as financially successful for us as our Tucson resort, it was a key to our evolution. It also allowed us to do something that would have been impossible without a second resort: Lenox transformed Canyon Ranch into a national brand.

Best Spa times two

Here's how quickly it happened. In 1990, *Condé Nast Traveler* magazine created a new category for "Best Spa." That first year, Tucson won. The second year of the award, Lenox won—and it had been open for only one full year. We had arrived! And by then, so had all sorts of people who wanted to talk to us about extending "the Canyon Ranch brand." Regularly at both resorts, we would see people walking around with cameras and notepads. They weren't taking vacation snapshots; they were making notes so they could keep up with the gold standard for the wellness industry. In a way, it was flattering.

Brand? What's that?

Jerry and I had never thought about building a brand. We had thought about building a successful business, of course.

But struggle as we might with money, we always looked beyond it. Canyon Ranch was meant to be a mission-driven business, which would allow us to take care of our employees and extend our vision of wellness to a larger community that couldn't afford to stay at our resort. We weren't interested in being a "brand," whatever that was.

People kept talking to us about it, though. One of the first people was a good friend from New York who suggested that we launch a skin care line, because, he said, "People recognize and trust your brand."

I went to Enid. "What do you think? Do we have a brand? Should we 'brand' a skin care line?" Enid, as always, was the chastity belt of the Canyon Ranch mission.

"Sure we have a brand, but what does it mean on a skin care line?" she said. "If it doesn't deliver on the mission, we shouldn't do it."

She was a killjoy, but of course she was right. There was no medical or health care reason to put our name on a jar of some cream or lotion that someone else just developed generically. [When we finally did offer a Canyon Ranch skin care line in 2005, it was because two scientists from the University of Arizona came to us with a scientifically based and tested product. We felt that evidence and results made the product worthy of the Canyon Ranch name.]

But people kept coming out of the woodwork, offering us money, encouraging us to multiply and grow. The outsiders' estimates of the financial value of the Canyon Ranch name seemed to escalate with every new pitch.

Many of the people who came to us with business proposals had first come to the ranch as guests and now returned as believers with checkbooks. One of them was Richard Rainwater, a world-class financier. He came to Tucson in 1994 because a friend had given him a Canyon Ranch gift certificate that was close to expiring. He was expecting nothing more than a pleasant vacation, but he fell in love with the place. At the end of his stay, he made an appointment to talk. He was starting a new real estate investment trust called Crescent Real Estate Equities, and he thought Canyon Ranch would be a good fit. He offered to buy the real estate of the two properties and give Jerry and me a long-term management contract. I was polite but firm. "No thanks," I said. "We're not for sale."

The reach of the ranch

We weren't a hotel concept like the Four Seasons or the Ritz Carlton that someone could buy, operate and extend. Canyon Ranch was a very different animal. And it was hungry for everything we could give it. We were going nuts, managing our two properties, perfecting our operations and trying to do a little good in the larger world. There were new health and healing services to coordinate for our guests, and a full-blown spirituality program. Our original collaboration with professionals from the University of Arizona had led us to an ongoing relationship with its Health Sciences Center and medical school. We were helping support research projects and education through the Prevention & Public Health program, and the Mel and Enid Zuckerman College of Public Health was born as a result. We had similar collaborations with other medical institutions around the country.

We'd also taken a leadership role in the local community with projects like an Elder Camp research program for Tucson's seniors. We'd established a scholarship program for Pima County residents at the ranch because we knew we were priced too high for many of them to come, and we didn't want to deny our services to people with health issues and a real need for the benefits we had to offer. We started a similar program in Lenox and had invited thousands of our neighbors to spend weeks as our guests at the ranch in both locations.

But it was time to take stock and think about what was really left for us to do. Jerry and I had developed a routine of taking hikes in the mountains, just the two of us. I'd loved hiking the trails with the guests in the early days of Canyon Ranch, but as the years progressed, when I went out with them, they were so interested in talking to me that I lost the sense of peace in the wilderness. Sometimes, perhaps too often, I felt as though I was less Mel Zuckerman than Mr.

Canyon Ranch. My mind was buzzing all the time. My regular quiet hikes with Jerry up Mount Lemmon became a kind of sacred time for us to reflect about the business without the distractions of the office.

A hike up Mount Lemmon

On one of those hikes, in early fall '95, Jerry and I stopped at a lookout point to have a snack. "OK," I said to Jerry, "What do we do now? We're out of the woods in Tucson and in Lenox. Are we going to stop here, or are we willing to let this brand thing play out?"

We had gotten through the bad years. Other people might've looked down from the mountain, surveying all they'd accomplished, and decided it was time to rest. I was 67 then, but I'd never been able to step back and relax. The truth was, I still needed challenges to keep from getting bored. I was never an "operating guy." Jerry could keep himself happy playing with the numbers and the details, but I needed creative challenges. I was a developer, and developers need to build.

So we sketched out a 10-year plan. Lenox had taught us that the Canyon Ranch experience didn't have to be just an immersion at a beautiful resort. A weekend visit, even a single session with one of our professionals, could spark a desire for change, and help put someone on the path to wellness. There were many avenues for touching people, many ways and places where they could get, and absorb, the message we'd been working to spread for so many years. That's how we'd think about our "brand"—as a way to say: This is our philosophy. How can we extend its reach?

But reaching into the world with a big idea takes money. Lots of money. And we had nowhere near the kind of financial wherewithal we'd need for the plans we were sketching out. How would we do it?

We didn't have to wait long for a solution. Richard Rainwater and his wife Darla came back to the ranch in January 1996. Once again, a few days into his stay, Rainwater came to see me in my office. "You guys are the leading edge of a new industry that has relevance everywhere. You should be in every gateway city in America. And you do it like nobody else in the world. Our REIT would be honored to have you in our portfolio." He practically let us write our own deal.

Jerry and I began to think about what it would do for us to sell the real estate to the REIT. It was sounding more and more attractive. After all, REITs don't operate businesses; they take the real and hard assets and leave the operators in place. We liked the idea as a way to guarantee that we'd be secure financially and professionally while continuing to mind the Canyon Ranch mission. How did a 50-year management contract sound? That should take us at least through early retirement. By the time it expired I'd be 118 and Jerry would be 102.

The deal we negotiated included that 50-year management contract, with good incentives for the two of us to continue to operate the resorts. Rainwater's Crescent operation would have a 30% stake in all future Canyon Ranch ventures beyond the two existing immersion resorts. Jerry flew to San Diego where I was vacationing with the papers to sign. We closed the deal on July 4th weekend.

When the news hit the financial press, some misunderstood the transaction and thought that we were no longer in control of our business. In fact we were in total control, and our performance as "operators" from 1996 until 2001 was extremely good. We started to hit 85% and 90% occupancies and became more profitable. We shared profits with Crescent, and we became the highest return on investment in Crescent's portfolio. Our management fees, which were based on profitability, kept increasing. Everyone was happy.

The funds from Crescent allowed us to go into ventures like the Las Vegas SpaClub at The Venetian, which opened in 1999. Though we'd once sworn that we'd never set up shop in Las Vegas, the spa club became the model for many of our future ventures, where we brought our philosophy to a location and operated the property, but did not own the underlying real estate. After Lenox, we never bought another property, and every Canyon Ranch venture since Las Vegas has followed the same structure.

It has been a thrill to see my little Aha! Moment at the Oaks come to define excellence for the wellness industry. Whether guests encounter Canyon Ranch for a week or for just an hour with one of our body workers, they come in contact with at least one person who will encourage them to think about improving their lives.

We did have some ventures that didn't take off. One of them was the idea of Canyon Ranch cruise ships. I loved the idea of a Canyon Ranch at Sea, a fully dedicated spa and wellness ship, where everything that was available to the guests at our immersion resorts would be available, plus exotic ports of call. I spent three years working on the concept, and we were ready to start building the ships until 9/11 put that idea to rest. (But maybe not forever.) In 2003, we announced that we would be operating a Canyon Ranch Living Miami Beach project, a 500-unit hotel and condo resort, to be built in the heart of Miami Beach on 700 feet of pristine beach. When that news hit the wire, it seemed like a marquee moment for the Canyon Ranch brand. Almost overnight, we were sought out by developers all over the country who wanted to bring us to their resorts, hotels and residential developments because of the added value our lifestyle experience and brand brought to their projects.

We thought hard about how to do this. In January 2005, at Crescent's behest, we jumped in, as usual, with both feet. We restructured the company's ownership and dramatically increased our debt so that we could take on opportunities that had emerged since we had announced the Miami deal. In the process, everything became 52% Canyon Ranch and 48% Crescent.

We were back in debt and thinking big. Within two years of the Miami Beach announcement, we had signed contracts to operate and be the brand name on projects in the Washington, D.C., area, in Chicago, in Costa Rica, Cabo San Lucas and Scottsdale, Arizona. Other developers were knocking at our door. The total value of these projects was in excess of $4 billion. Our brand fees on just three of these projects would have paid off all our newly incurred debt and allowed us to seek further opportunities. Our new development division at one time was evaluating 11 projects, knowing that at most we could do seven in the following 10 years. We were flying high.

And by now, you have probably guessed the rest of the story. The boom turned to bust, and we crashed into the Great Recession of the last few years. After two years of work in the development process of these projects, every single one of them disappeared from our screen.

So in 2010, we were once again steeped in debt, struggling with occupancies and cash flow—yet extremely confident about Canyon Ranch's future.

By now you've seen the pattern, and so have I. Just as things seem to be swimming along, a financial catastrophe strikes, or I get a new idea, or entertain a proposition that amounts to doubling down on our risk. I know. I know. I should be satisfied with all that we've accomplished so far, and let the future take care of itself. But I can't. At 82, I'm still too restless for that, and still driven by our mission to change lives for the better.

In the corner of my eye, just within my field of vision, I see the future of Canyon Ranch. It might be international, or even global in its reach. I don't know the details, but I do know the mission and the vision: reaching out for the power of possibility.

Mukta Mel

—————◆—————

I t's fascinating to me, reflecting as I write, that a person so beset by stress and striving could create spaces where so many could experience powerful moments of joy and find both physical and spiritual healing. It's a paradox that I'll try to explain with the story of "Mukta Mel."

After I left Ojai in April 1978 I often thought about my time there. Ojai was then considered a "spiritual" community, whatever that meant. I remember that staff members had told me of visits to Ojai by a spiritual guru by the name of Swami Muktananda who held "spiritual" seminars in the hills behind Ojai. They used to come to work the next day glowing in the "enlightenment" of this spiritual leader. Unfortunately, they could never really explain exactly what the swami had done for them, but it was clear he had offered something important, some kind of spiritual wisdom well worth attaining.

I thought about the swami from time to time, and he resurfaced in my mind in 1980, when I decided to excavate behind an old mesquite tree in a lovely lawn area behind the clubhouse and near the creek bed. I had always felt the area was special, a place for reflection. I thought I'd build an amphitheater there for evening outdoor lectures where guests and staff could come together at nightfall to learn and listen. I could see it clearly, a guest lecturer sharing his or expertise, or a staff member giving a talk, while the guests, tired and relaxed after a busy day on the ranch, would soak it all in.

Then I had an epiphany. This amphitheater, in the ancient, magical shadow of the mesquite, wouldn't just be an outdoor lecture hall, but would also be a space for sacred, spiritual gatherings. And someday, wise and liberated from earthly desire—I would sit at the center. I couldn't really see myself as a swami. No, I would be Mukta Mel, wizened and old, wearing a long, flowing robe, with a flower garland around my neck, and have long gray hair and a long white beard. I'd be 90, entering the sixth 18-year chai cycle of my life. In the Jewish tradition, chai is a powerful number. Our toast, "L'chaim!" means "to life," and every new 18-year cycle represents another chance for a renewal of the soul and spirit. I figured that I blew my first two chai cycles—18 years as an introvert, the next 18 becoming an anxious adult. And though I'd started the ranch in the middle of my third cycle, I didn't think it very likely I'd get to spiritual maturity and enlightenment much before the sixth, when I'd be a wise man in long red robes chanting "Om" while my disciples sat in a circle at my feet and nodded. Having achieved great wisdom, I would send my soul off into space, on the spiritual journey of a lifetime. It was a beautiful, inspiring vision, and I almost believed it.

But suddenly a very loud voice in my head said, "Hey guy! Who are you kidding? There's nothing spiritual about you! Your mind is consumed with day-to-day noise. You aren't going to be anything like a spiritual guru if you keep fighting the battles of everyday life." Then, another voice chimed in. "You know, Mel," it said soothingly, "if you seek your deepest spiritual self, you could become Mukta Mel, completing the spiritual journey by your sixth chai cycle. Focus on goodness, on purpose, on your desire to help others, on your original goal of making the planet a better, healthier place to live." When my two selves get into an argument, my head gets to be a pretty noisy neighborhood.

I kept moving ahead with the idea. I was working on my chanting skills, and the backhoes were purring. But with the first scrape of the ground in my sacred spot, water came surging up. Stop the shovels! The tree was too close to the creek and the water table was too shallow. I could put in my amphitheater, but it would cost me 50 times more than I had expected, and we just couldn't afford to do it. I had to abandon the whole idea. There went the vision of Mukta Mel.

No robes. No flower garland. No liberation from striving and strife. I'd have to keep battling to find my own peace, spirituality and joy.

As Canyon Ranch has blossomed, I have watched as more and more guests enter into a deeper, different consciousness during their visits. They exercise their bodies hard, and in the process their spirits become softer and more receptive to joy in the universe. In many ways it is an extreme irony that I built a business that has enabled so many to find what has so often eluded me. I know that something important and deeply transforming happens to people during their time at the ranch. I see it, I hear it and I feel it every single day on every one of our properties. Our power to create and sustain positive change puts me in awe of what emanated from my own simple experience at the Oaks, where the ability to jog a mile and a half put me over the moon.

I still believe that the straightest, best route to wellness includes a lot of exercise, but I know that exercise alone won't bring you to spiritual balance. Spirituality, after all, is a journey without a destination, just as perfection is. That has been an important lesson for a perfectionist like me, who has enormous difficulty letting things be, living with the imperfect or the half-achieved vision. I am not a religious person, but I can't deny God's existence either, because I think and speak about a higher power directing me to create Canyon Ranch and electing me to shepherd it. I know these words sound funny coming from someone who has spent pages and pages documenting financial and personal struggles to overcome the odds. But the mission itself has driven me. Honest and truly.

Sometimes I think that Enid and I deluded ourselves by thinking that Canyon Ranch was all about us, and selfishly wanting to maintain our own well-being. How quickly I have always let go of the dream that might have given me the most inner peace and let the entrepreneur take over again! Maybe the plan was never for me to be at peace. Or, maybe our original plan was pure rationalization. I feel lucky because so many go through so much of life without finding real meaning. Enid and I have been very lucky indeed. Sometimes, we struggle. Are we Canyon Ranch? Or is Canyon Ranch us? Who knows? In our lifetimes we are one and the same, and inseparable. We know that there is a long, successful future for Canyon Ranch without us. We rejoice in wondering what the future holds for the fantasy we conceived on that long drive back from Ojai to Tucson in 1978. Our future, our sense of spirituality, is at rest within the walls of Canyon Ranch. Mukta Mel still whispers to me when I am in the mood to listen, guiding me and helping me stay true to my own spiritual mission: creating a space for health and healing for others in need.

With lots of help from supportive family and insightful friends at Canyon Ranch, I have become more willing to tap into things that are larger and more important than the moment. I've found a lot of satisfaction in working to bring better health to many through public health, education about disease prevention and working with heart-centered charities like Dream Street, which supports kids living with cancer and other life-threatening diseases. Time with my wife, my grandkids and my children connects me to that "something larger" too.

Now, when challenges come along—in business, to my health, within my family and close circle of friends—I try to breathe deeply and train my eye to a longer perspective. It still isn't easy for me to keep my cool or my balance, but those occasional private visits from Mukta Mel keep me focused on the long view of my life and mission.

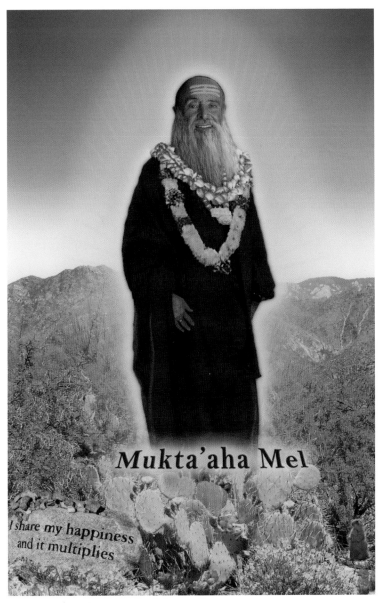

Mukta'aha Mel

I share my happiness
and it multiplies

Courtesy of Jim Levin

I've taken a great deal of comfort and guidance from this passage in that long ago astrological reading from Nancy Bissell, written in 1980, just at the dawn of Canyon Ranch.

"Success is one of the main themes of this chart. There is a potential for power and far-reaching influence, status, wealth and achievement. Notice, however, that the twelfth house in your wheel is occupied by three planets: this indicates that there could be some kind of ironic counterpart to all this, some way in which the concept of success is more complex and subtle than it first appears.

"For the twelfth is the house of compassion, and service, and spiritual responsibility. In some way the idea of sacrifice is present. Perhaps you will never feel adequately recognized for your accomplishments; or maybe you recognize on some deeper lever that material success itself will never bring you a true sense of personal satisfaction but that some other more profound area must be explored, centered around the idea of service.

"Your experiences in the first part of your life, in their fiery intensity, continue to teach you that real success has to do with reaching in with the same boldness as your reaching out. Attunement to your inner nature provides the equilibrium and peace of mind that lies at the center of your restless search. Set your goals as high as your imagination will allow. You will receive hidden support from the universal forces (Jupiter in Aries in the twelfth), and cannot possibly go wrong.

The Take Away

———◆·◆·◆———

We are at the end of my story, a story of how one chaotic and crazy guy turned his whole life around. My story is unusual, but it need not be unique.

If all this could happen to me, it could happen to you. At 50 years old, I had nothing in my favor, other than the stars and the moons. I was an asthmatic, lonely kid, grown into a driven man who soaked up stress like a dry sponge. Magically, I found my way to Ojai, at precisely the right moment in my life for an Aha! Moment.

But it is not only about the moment. It is also about being ready to make a change. It would not have mattered one whit if I had gone to the Oaks, met Karma Kientzler, or if Enid had mentioned to me her wacky idea about opening a "fat farm" in Tucson, if I had not been ready to change.

Aha! Moments are chance encounters that come to the receptive mind and soul.

This can be your Aha! Moment if you let it. Chances are you're not nearly as imperfect, restless and irrational as I am. But even if you are, I hope you've gotten the message of this book. Change starts with a decision. It's impartial—it doesn't really care what road brought you to its door or how badly you've screwed up. Change is about this moment. So make one small decision right now to choose health. Get your body moving every day. Put gorgeous vegetables on your plate. Try to find joy and give joy every day. Do it again, and again, and again. And keep going.

Truth be told, most of us know the things we should be doing to live more healthfully, but today you have the opportunity to close the gap between what you know and what you do. Connect the dots. That's what we do at Canyon Ranch.

But even with as much information as is available, not everyone knows how to take the first step. It's not my way to leave you on the cusp of change without offering some guidance. To help you take your next steps, I'm working on a short companion handbook. In it, I have attempted to cover the basics required to prevent disease, maintain good health, and to age with optimal physical and mental functioning.

Think about this: At age 40, my biological "clock" read that I was living in the body of a 65- to 70-year-old man. Twenty-five years later, at age 65, the same type of test concluded that I now had the body of a man 20 to 25 years younger than my chronological age. By embracing a healthy lifestyle, I had reset my "clock" back 20 to 25 years. Decades of an interesting, energetic life might have been denied to me had I not made a commitment to change. It's powerful stuff, but it isn't magic. And if I could do it, flawed, restless and irrational as I am—so can you.

Life is a wonderful gift, and with hope, purpose and perseverance, you can accomplish almost anything. The power of possibility resides in each of us. I wish you great success on your journey toward a healthy life.

ACKNOWLEDGMENTS

————◆•◉•◆————

To my late parents, Shirley and Norman Zuckerman. To my father for his humility, empathy and overall humanity. His life—and his death—each in its own way was the catalyst for creating Canyon Ranch.

And to my mother, who instilled in me the drive for perfection and achievement. My career and my life are testaments to her guidance and perseverance.

To my children, Jay and Amy, and to my grandchildren and great-grandchildren. I cherish my family. Their lives inspire me, and give me my reason for living.

To Jerry Cohen, my dear friend and partner, and often my alter ego. An operating genius who has shared with me the struggles and crises of the last 30 years. Thank you, Jerry, for allowing me to achieve what would have been impossible without you.

To Karma Kientzler, who 32 years ago looked at an unhappy

and dangerously unhealthy guy and introduced him to a force he never before encountered: the power of possibility. To this day, Karma continues as a forceful energy in my well-being and in the evolution of Canyon Ranch.

To my good friend and associate for more than 30 years, John Campisano. Our personal and professional relationship began in the home building business. When I decided to build Canyon Ranch, it was John's inspirational and architectural genius that enabled me to turn a dilapidated dude ranch in Tucson into a world-renowned resort.

To the late Andy Arena, a friend and colleague who was a source of support for me during my most difficult days.

To a few of the people who, during the early years of the ranch, were instrumental in adding new dimension to the Canyon Ranch vision: Thank you, Jeanne Jones, Phyllis Hochman and Deborah Morris Coryell. A very special thanks to Dan Baker whose special contributions in the mid '80s defined our behavioral/life management programs and established the Life Enhancement Center. Over the last 22 years, the LEC has become the premier lifestyle change program in the world.

To the extraordinary physicians who brought their passion and talent and created the Canyon Ranch brand of integrated medicine. To Dr. Andrew Weil, in particular, for opening me up to the frontiers of medicine beyond Western medicine. And to Dr. Phil Eichling, and to our corporate medical director, Dr. Mark Liponis. Thank you all for bringing your professional guidance, creativity and special energies to the development of unique and integrated medical programming.

To the thousands of dedicated staff at every level, who over the years believed in our mission and in our vision, and committed themselves with us on the journey to perfection. Simply put, without their genuine caring for our guests, and their extraordinary professionalism, Canyon Ranch would not be deserving of the reputation it enjoys.

To our Canyon Ranch guests for helping us evolve. Their input and insights have made them our most important asset. Our guests have been crucial to creating the "Canyon Ranch Experience."

And, though it would take an entire book to list them all by name, I would like to acknowledge and thank all our personal friends, our professional supporters and advisors, and our many longtime guests whose affection and intelligence have meant so much to Enid and to me over the years.

A great debt of thanks to my assistant, Kathy Tolzman. Her unflappable efficiency and perseverance through this entire process allowed the project to keep humming through to completion. And to our editor, Donna Frazier Glynn, for her graceful editing and the serenity she brought to the effort.

A special heartfelt thanks to my co-author, Louisa Kasdon, for her skill, good humor and patience, and for arguing with me through every single sentence, and for her commitment to helping me tell my story in my own words.

– *Mel Zuckerman, 2010*

DEDICATION AND
ACKNOWLEDGMENTS

———◆•◆•◆———

To my mother and father, Muriel and Dr. S. Charles Kasdon, who shaped me with their values, their humor and their imagination.

To my amazing daughters, Katie Ellias and Evi Ellias, for their judgment and love.

And to my husband, Michael, for giving me new wings.

It has been my great honor to work with Mel Zuckerman and to share his story with our readers. I thank him for his patience, unflagging energy and exceptional (and occasionally irascible) quest for perfection. I also thank Enid Zuckerman, who kept us both honest in the process. She was a candid and critical reader throughout and was as central to this effort as she was to the saga of Canyon Ranch.

I thank the many professionals at Canyon Ranch who generously offered their recollections of Canyon Ranch's early days and gave me the grounding to understand how the ranch has matured. Although there are many, a special debt to Jerry Cohen, who believed that this project was worth the time it took. And to Karma Kientzler, who filled in so many important details.

A huge helping of thanks to Kathy Tolzman, Mel's extraordinary assistant, for keeping us out of eternal version hell, and for always reminding me that we were indeed making progress.

Many thanks to Donna Frazier Glynn, our editor, and to Sheri Gordon, our copy editor.

And to my many fellow guests at Canyon Ranch over the years, who sat with me at the Captain's Table, chatted with me on the morning walks and willingly traded their intimate experiences with me. When I doubted, their stories of hope and transformation nudged me back on the path.

– Louisa Kasdon, 2010